Promoting Independence and Ac

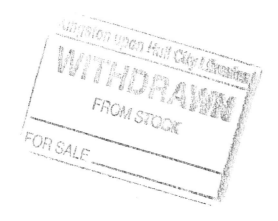

Note

Health care practice and knowledge are constantly changing and developing as new research and treatments, changes in procedures, drugs and equipment become available.

The author and publishers have, as far as is possible, taken care to confirm that the information complies with the latest standards of practice and legislation.

This book acts as a guide to the range of available options. Treatments, products, equipment and organisations named within this book do not imply endorsement of a particular product; nor does omission indicate disapproval. Certain equipment and adaptations are zero rated for Value Added Tax (VAT).

Neither the author nor the publisher can accept legal responsibility for personal injury, or any other damage, or loss arising from the use of any equipment; or following any course of action stated herein including misuse of the information provided in this book. Such remedies must be sought from the manufacturers of the equipment, or the suppliers of any services concerned.

Promoting Independence and Activity in Older People

Julie I. Swann

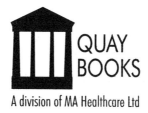

QUAY
BOOKS

A division of MA Healthcare Ltd

Quay Books Division, MA Healthcare Ltd, St Jude's Church, Dulwich Road, London
SE24 0PB

British Library Cataloguing-in-Publication Data
A catalogue record is available for this book

ISBN-10: 1 85642 334 4
ISBN-13: 978 1 85642 334 2

Printed by Athenaeum Press Ltd, Dukesway, Team Valley, Gateshead, SE11 0PZ

Contents

Part 4
Supporting individuals with their personal care needs

Part 5
Supporting individuals in dressing

Part 6
Helping individuals to eat and drink

Part 7
Continence management

Part 8
Recreational activities

Contents

Part 12
The future

Preface

This book is about helping older people achieve independence. The emphasis throughout is on personal care: finding the best way to help people maintain their level of independence and stay active for as long as possible.

Although it focuses on those who are mainly in residential care settings, the content is relevant to problems that can occur at any age and in any setting.

Carers will find this practical approach particularly useful in helping them in their important role of enabling people to become more independent and to manage tasks more easily.

The book is based upon articles written in the *International Journal of Therapy and Rehabilitation* in 2006 and for the practical series in Residential and Nursing Care, published between 2004 and 2007.

This book can be read in its entirety or used as a reference source when problems arise. Each part is separate, but several major themes emerge.

Part 1 describes the changes that occur due to ageing. The effect of ageing on cognitive abilities and physical function is described and the impact of moving into a care home setting is explored.

Part 2 considers environmental barriers that can affect people with cognitive and physically problems and prevent their full participation in society.

Part 3 outlines the importance of continuous assessment. Different techniques that can be used to make tasks easier, and the use of assistive devices to overcome barriers are discussed.

Parts 4–7 concentrate on supporting individuals with personal care activities, including ways in which tasks can be simplified, or adaptations and assistive devices used. Topics include: personal hygiene, washing bodies, bathing, showering, dressing difficulties including cognitive problems, eating and drinking problems, toileting and urinary incontinence.

Part 8 concentrates on leisure and recreation. In addition to providing basic care, it is an integral part of a care home's philosophy to provide a varied programme of optional activities for residents, and it is also part of the Care Home for Older People National Minimum Standards 12 to 15. Suggestions are provided for group and individual activities to include in programmes, ranging from gardening to pampering sessions.

Part 9 is about keeping mobile. Mobility problems and the correct use of mobility appliances are discussed, and movement to music is outlined.

Part 10 describes three of the major medical conditions: strokes, Parkinsonism and multiple sclerosis. These chapters explain how such conditions affect the body, and how carers can help to overcome problems of mobility and daily living.

Part 11 introduces the rehabilitation team and some specialised techniques that traditional and complementary therapists use and encourages carers to work with therapists, to facilitate and maintain movement patterns.

The final part of the book explores the Internet and computers, discussing the ways in which technology can shape the care sector and future of care homes.

Many chapters contain information for candidates who are taking, or have taken, S/NVQs in Care. Although this book is primarily intended for care staff and managers within a care home, other readers will find the content useful, in particular: students and practitioners within the caring professions; people who have difficulties with activities of daily living and mobility; housing associations; and providers of care in the community.

Julie I. Swann
Independent Occupational Therapist
April 2007

PART I

Transitions

CHAPTER I

The journey into care

Life is full of changes; everyone experiences varying emotional reactions to these at different stages in life. One of the most traumatic periods occurs when a person needs to move from living in their own home into a care home. This decision is not like choosing to move house; it is much more profound, as it means moving into a totally different lifestyle. Moving into care can be welcome, as it may bring an end to household responsibilities, with the provision of increased assistance at hand and companionship. Choosing a residential or nursing home can be a very daunting experience for older people as well for their relatives or friends. With a positive approach, it is possible to minimise any negative impact of this transition.

Care in the community

Successive governments have emphasised the value of helping people to remain within their own homes rather than being hospitalised or moving into care. Community Care initiatives in the 1990s focused on well-integrated coordinated health and social care services from a myriad of different providers. Responsibility for intensive assessments and management of care services for people with complex needs fell to Social Services Departments. In recent years, many different and effective services have emerged to support this philosophy, including:

- Intensive care worker support within a person's own home. Care is now available up to 24/7 over 365 days, including night attendance, provided by statutory services or privately.
- Home care organisations that provide help with personal tasks, domestic chores, shopping and home maintenance. They can provide intensive personal care, including teams of 'live-in' carers.
- Direct payments to fund care arrangements emerging as a method of enhancing people's independence and choice.
- Expansion of community health services and the increasingly important role of primary care.

■ Continued progress in the number and range of different forms of assistive equipment and adaptations.

■ Creative use of residential facilities for short-term breaks, respite and inter-mediate care.

■ Development of resource or community care centres with support services, all located in one place.

■ Emergence and development of technology, such as telecare.

Care in the community packages support people with disabilities, poor physical health or frailty by using informal and formal carers. This trend is likely to continue as new organisational forms emerge within local govern-ments and their health partners. Social Care departments are replacing Social Services with major developments of joint teams with health and other col-leagues.

The evidence shows that community care initiatives have been success-ful. Community Care Statistics (2005) provides information on residential and nursing care placements funded by Councils with Social Services Responsi-bilities (CSSRs). Their data relate to the type of care, sector, client group, stay and age for supported residents in England (as at 31 March 2005). Sixty per cent of supported residents were in independent residential care homes, 28% in independent nursing homes and 10% in CSSR staffed homes. This figure includes 18% 'out of area' placements. The number of supported residents in CSSRs and independent residential and nursing homes, including unstaffed homes, decreased to 267,200, a fall of 10,700 (4%) on the previous year. The majority of people who enter a care environment are over 65 years old (Com-munity Care Statistics, 2005).

Whilst the prevailing philosophy concerning good care for individuals in this country is encapsulated in the phrase 'Care in the Community', some people will always need a care home, and this can be seen as a positive choice.

The need for residential care

People generally choose to live within their own home environment but, for some, it is not possible to achieve or maintain completely independent living. Despite the rapid expansion of services promoting care in the community, there are times when it is no longer feasible for people to stay in their own homes. This may be because of sudden incapacity, illness of main carers or a gradual decline in their own level of abilities. Care arrangements may no longer meet needs; for example, carers may be unable to provide the level of physical help, or they may themselves be unable to cope (perhaps because of their own ill health). Alternatively, it may be that the intensity of care required is not available within a community setting. These and many other factors can trigger the need to move into a care home. This may happen during a period of crisis rather than in a planned and coordinated fashion. The following case studies are true, but the names have been changed.

Case study

Elsie had looked after her husband, John, aged 63, since he had a severe stroke. With the provision of equipment, including a hoist, alterations to the access of their home and a level-access shower, she was able to care for him, with support from the District Nurses and her family. Elsie died suddenly and John moved into residential care.

Many people in care suffer from dementia, but it is possible to provide support at home for many years, particularly if people are mobile and only require prompts and assistance with complex tasks aided by 'smart' technology (Chapter 34). However, profiles of residents in care indicate that dementia figures prominently in the reason for admission. Managing people in the community can be particularly complex and clear risk assessments need to take place, with contingency plans written into the care package.

Case study

Jane gradually became more forgetful and her brother Frank had noticed she kept burning food and could not complete any household tasks. Her GP diagnosed dementia. When getting dressed, she put items on the wrong part of her body. Frank simply provided prompts in a non-critical way and followed her around to ensure that she was not in any danger. Gas appliances were changed to electric to reduce the risk of accidents if she inadvertently left the cooker or fire on. Frank went to the local shop for the daily groceries and the supermarket delivered bulk shopping. One day, Frank fell, and Jane did not know what to do; she could not work out how to use the phone. She covered him up with a blanket. Three days later a neighbour called round. Jane said that Frank was having a nap. Frank had died of a heart attack. Jane was admitted to a residential home specialising in dementia care.

As people age, abilities tend to decline; the main effects of ageing are discussed in Chapter 2. A sudden illness, a fall, or worsening of a progressive medical condition can precipitate a period of hospital stay. Levels of independence may not return sufficiently for safe discharge home, and may necessitate transfer into residential or nursing home care.

Case study

Eddie, a frail widower, aged 91, suffered from low blood pressure and had a history of falling. He was admitted to hospital with arrhythmia. After a pacemaker was inserted, it was felt to be in his best interests if he moved into residential care.

Many young people live in care homes, including homes that cater for the under 50s. For some, transition into independent living as an adult may be impossible and this is therefore a permanent move. Admission may be temporary until funds are available for adaptations to be made to property, or indeed until single-storey accommodation and a full package of care is funded.

Case study

Simon, aged 20, was involved in a fight and sustained brain trauma, resulting in a brain haemorrhage causing left sided hemiplegia. After four months of hospital care, he moved into a nursing home for two years until funding was provided through the Criminal Injuries Compensation Board for accommodation and care.

John, aged 28, suffered major brain injuries in a car accident. On discharge from hospital he moved into a nursing home.

Taking a decision to move into care

People often move home to better their living environment or to downsize to release capital, and this is generally a positive choice. Moving home is a stressful experience, comparable with the levels of stress experienced in other major life-changing events, such as bereavement or divorce; moving into residential

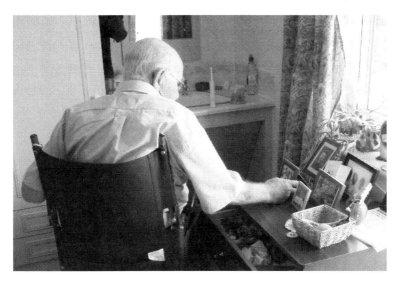

Time to reflect and reminisce (© NRC 2006).

care is equally stressful. In addition to the upheaval associated with the move, people may be entering an unknown environment. There can be a deep sense of loss of personal autonomy and control over aspects of daily living and personal tasks. New residents experience not only a change of location and environment but also a sense of loss of control over aspects of life that they had hitherto taken for granted. Routines developed over years are completely disrupted. Dependency on others, often strangers, occurs to manage personal tasks they had previously managed independently and privately for many years.

Some people are admitted to care during a personal crisis, such as the loss of a carer or an illness necessitating hospital care. These other traumas have to be dealt with in addition to adjusting to the emotions aroused when moving into care. Admission to care can therefore be overlaid with traumatic feelings, which are shared by carers and family members, who are themselves adjusting to the changed situation. There may also be feelings of inadequacy and guilt as carers reproach themselves for their inability to help the individual stay at home. There can be positive and negative changes of roles within a family when one member of the family enters a care home.

Easing the transition

Social Services has a statutory duty to assess eligibility for residential or nursing home care and have to complete assessments in a given time. However, there can be delays of weeks or even months whilst funding is arranged, particularly when a person is admitted to hospital while away from their home. A delay in admission can result in distress and a 'bed blockage' on an acute ward for the hospital. For relatives, delay can mean that the chosen room in the ideal local home is lost and another home has to be considered. Meanwhile, their relative is occupying a hospital bed, often sharing a ward with other people who are very ill.

Entering care should be tailored to meet an individual's unique needs, and a thorough assessment is essential. Aubrey-Fletcher (2002) looked at ways in which a resident's transition from their own accommodation into a care home can be facilitated. She described how this life-changing decision can be a traumatic experience for the older person and their family, and that the situation can be eased with careful planning, guidance and support. Davies and Nolan (2004) collected data in 37 semi-structured interviews involving 48 people who had assisted a close relative to move to a nursing home. Their findings suggest that health and social care professionals have enormous potential to influence the resident's and relatives' experiences of nursing home entry. The experiences were enhanced if family carers worked in partnership with care staff to ease the transition. One factor that influences transition is the degree of control that individuals believe they have over their own actions, personal circumstances and life management.

Good information

When a decision is made to move into a care home, there are two main tasks: to find a home that is suitable and to obtain funding. Neither of these tasks is easy and both are time-consuming. Lists of care homes are available from Social Services and the hospital discharge liaison/coordinator. The Commission for Social Care Inspection (CSCI) web site (http://www.csci.org.uk/) provides a UK directory of homes within a 5 to 50 mile radius of a given postcode and provides full inspection reports of individual homes. Several other web sites can also help locate care homes: for example, Bettercaring (http://www.bettercaring.co.uk/), the Care Directory (http://www.nursing-home-directory.co.uk/) and Registered Nursing Home Association (http://www.rnha.co.uk/).

A prospective resident may never have visited a care home. Relatives, friends or the potential resident may have previously visited someone in a care home and gained a positive or negative impression. Although personal recommendation is useful, and often acted upon, it is to be remembered that everyone has different tastes and needs and what suits one person may not suit another.

Having a look first

No one would dream of buying a house or renting a property without having a good look around first. Whenever possible, the potential resident and family or other significant people should visit the care home before placement. Visiting at different times of the day certainly provides a more rounded opinion. UK Nursing Homes Directory (2002) (`http://www.ucarewecare.com/`) advises people to 'Treat your visit as if you were buying a house and trust your feelings', and lists 12 questions to consider when choosing a care home:

1. How regularly do doctors visit the nursing home?
2. Does the home cater for nursing as well as residential care? This would be preferable to moving again a later date if necessary.
3. Do the homes retain their key staff? A long-term relationship between staff and residents is important.
4. Does each home on your shortlist have space available at the time of expected admission?
5. Does the home have a care plan or adopt a particular philosophy?
6. What emphasis does the home give to caring for the resident?
7. What makes this particular home different from others you have enquired about?
8. Does the home offer any special activities that will interest your loved one?
9. Does the geographical location make visiting possible at any time by family and friends? Regular visits are the best way to make sure that your loved one does well.
10. Are there sufficient local transport options available?
11. Are residents' religious denominations and cultural needs catered for?
12. Are special dietary requirements catered for?

Many factors influence choice of a home including the location, nearness to community facilities, word of mouth, personal experience of the care home, availability of beds, physical layout and access to local facilities. The location and facilities of the home are important, but equal, if not more, weight is placed on other factors: for example, the way staff approach the potential resident and their general interaction with other residents in the home. This aspect is very significant, as a home may be in pristine condition and compliant with all the CSCI standards, but does not give a 'feel good' factor to the prospective resident.

Settling in

Residents need time to settle in and to establish their own routines. It is important to let routines continue and to be sensitive to the individual's needs. Some habits are difficult to change: for example, one resident turned off all the lights and unplugged the TV sockets before he went to bed, thus leaving the home in total darkness. Another resident waited at the front door every day at 4:00 p.m., as this was the time her children had returned home from school. Knowledge of a resident's previous lifestyle and habits will help to enable care staff to understand and adjust to individual idiosyncrasies, and this information should be passed on. Relatives, friends, former carers and care agencies are the best sources of information, particularly if the resident is not a good communicator.

Many people will need to adjust to living with others in a more communal social setting. There has to be an adjustment to the prevailing social norms within the care home, getting to know other people and fitting into new routines: for example, meal times and going to bed.

Carers' needs

But what of the people who are left at home in the community when a person moves into a care home? It can be upsetting for relatives or for a long-term partner when saying goodnight before returning alone to a house that is now empty. Staff should be aware of this need and take appropriate steps to engage relatives, partners or friends in the ongoing care of individuals and any activities they participate in. Several homes offer activities that the local community and families and people living in the local community can become involved with, such as quiz events, musical nights or day trips. It can also be quite distressing to visit relatives when they are deteriorating. It is to the credit of many homes that some relatives maintain contact with the care home after their loved one has passed away.

Conclusion

Moving into a care home is one of the most stressful transitions that an individual will ever face. It can signify the end of an independent lifestyle and the start of communal living with many other people, perhaps after years of living alone independently since a partner died. For some residents, perhaps years of social isolation and deprivation are exchanged for a better, happier and safer living arrangement. Towards the end of natural life there may well be some degree of dependency and it can, for some people, become very difficult to live supported in the community.

A care home can meet some individual needs more effectively and provide a better quality of life. With proper planning and forethought, it is possible to adopt a positive approach to this event. All staff involved can help smooth the transition into a care home and make the process of entering and experiencing residential care as comfortable and happy as possible.

Key points

- Care in the community has been a positive and successful development.
- Assessment is essential before any admission to ensure appropriate placement.
- Moving into a care home can be very stressful.
- With proper arrangements in place, it is possible to minimise the trauma of admission.
- Staff from all sectors need to work together to ease the transition process.
- Residents need time to adjust to their new living arrangements.

CHAPTER 2

Ageing

Age brings on many changes, including the positive benefit of experience and the wisdom to make better judgements; yet ageing also brings about biological changes. Although wrinkles and grey hair are inevitable age-related changes, many alterations to bones and muscles occur because they are simply not used often enough. Evidence indicates that increasing activity improves health and reduces the risk of disability and chronic disease (Better Health Channel, 2006). Similarly, cognitive decline is less in people who engage more frequently in cognitively stimulating activities (Bosma *et al.*, 2002).

For all three lifestyle components (social, mental, and physical), Fratiglioni *et al.* (2004) suggest that when people have an active and socially integrated lifestyle there is a beneficial effect on cognition and a protective effect against dementia. The normal ageing process affects both physical function and cognitive abilities.

Physical function

Ageing may impose restrictions on physical activities, particularly strenuous tasks, within a home environment. Orthopaedic problems occur due to natural wear and tear and suppleness is reduced. Distance senses – sight and hearing – become progressively worse, with higher frequency noises during conversations becoming difficult to hear. Proximal senses, i.e. touch, are increasingly relied upon. Many older people complain of pain in their legs; this is partially due to ischaemia caused by poor circulation (intermittent claudication), which can result in painful cramps. Conversely, pain due to trauma can be minimal or even absent in the older person. Even a fracture of the neck of the femur may cause only slight discomfort, evidenced by a disinclination to walk or a slightly abnormal gait pattern. Age-related problems can cause individuals to start to have falls.

The National Minimum Care Standards (Department of Health, 2002a) stipulate that care homes must make an assessment of the resident's history of falling, unless this has been carried out prior to admission into care. Many measures can be taken by care homes to reduce the risks of a fall, including removal of hazards, ensuring resident's vision is checked regularly, providing a healthy diet and monitoring the effects of medication, as all these factors can increase the risk of falling. The National Institute for Health and Clinical Excellence (NICE) (2004) has produced a free information booklet on falls for older people, their families and carers (`http://www.nice.org.uk/guidance/CG21/publicinfo/pdf/English`); printed copies can be ordered via NICE's web site.

Cognitive function

Working memory and episodic memory are terms that refer to the structures and processes used to temporarily store and manipulate information received by all of the senses. The process used to 'hold on' to small bits of recently learned information, for example a telephone number, is called working memory or immediate memory. Episodic memory is the memory of an event or an 'episode' of a recent or remote event, like remembering what you did today (University of California Regents, 2006). The ability to recall new events or facts tends to gradually decline, which results in the names of objects and people being easily forgotten. This reduces the ability to remember the details of events and to cope with the complexities of life.

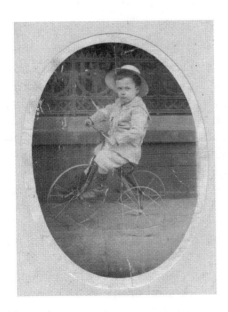 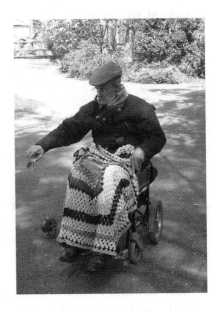

Bill at the ages of 3 and 93 (© Julie Swann 2007).

Braver *et al.* (2001) carried out an extensive literature search on cognitive functioning in healthy ageing people. Their findings 'suggested that older adults display deficits in multiple different cognitive domains, episodic memory, working memory, inhibition, attention and "executive" functions'. Problems with visuo-spatial tasks may also occur but all of these are part of the normal ageing process.

Yet, on the positive side, the vocabulary and verbal reasoning (semantic knowledge and memory) of older people often remains unchanged, or may improve during the ageing process. These processes, termed procedural memory, are the long-term memory of skills, the 'how to do' knowledge. This can be basic simple stimulus–response pairing or more extensive patterns of behaviour learnt over time.

Reminiscence of memory for emotional events is maintained with age. This explains why people can often recount and enhance tales of years gone by, and remember recipes and songs, but forget where they have put their glasses or dentures. Some societies revere older people and elder statespersons can have a high social standing. This is less so in today's consumer-driven, rapid progress, high-technology societies.

Dementia

All older adults experience a mild decline in specific areas of cognition. The term 'dementia' is used to describe a clinical syndrome encompassing progressive impairments in memory, abstract thought and judgement (executive functioning) and personality change. The Social Services Inspectorate (1996) estimated that 20% of people in the UK over the age of 80 and 6% over the age of 65 are affected by dementia. Over 750,000 people are affected by dementia in the UK, including around 18,000 people under the age of 65. Alzheimer's disease is the commonest form, making up 55% of all cases of dementia (Alzheimer's Society, 2004).

Problems and symptoms that can arise in people suffering from dementia, extracted from the University of California Regents (2006) web site, include:

- **Problems:**
  Executive functioning
  Language
  Working (immediate) memory
  Spatial memory
  Verbal memory

■ **Symptoms to look out for:**
Getting lost in familiar places
Constantly asking the same questions of staff
Odd or inappropriate behaviours
Forgetfulness of recent events
Repeated falls or loss of balance
Personality changes
Decline in planning and organisation
Changes in diet/eating habits
Alteration of personal hygiene
Increased apathy
Changes in language abilities, including comprehension

Physiological reasons for confusion

Physical problems, and the gradual emergence of cognitive problems, may simply be attributed to growing old. However, sometimes confusion may occur due to a symptom-less problem, like an infection, or powerful drugs causing a toxic confusional state. Symptoms of confusional states may arise abruptly over a few days. Accurate objective reporting of any noticeable changes is essential, particularly as medication may be the cause. It is therefore important to carry out a thorough assessment of short-term problems, as many cognitive problems, over and above slight forgetting, may be part of a treatable illness and need investigating.

Symptoms vary, and what is construed as 'normal' behaviour for one person may be totally out of character and therefore 'abnormal' for another person. This can make a diagnosis difficult for clinicians when deciding whether a decline is due to dementia, a physiological reason that is treatable or a psychological condition (excessive worry, depression, anxiety, etc.). Sometimes accelerated cognitive decline may not occur until certain events, such as a stroke, reach a threshold where the brain can no longer compensate for damage.

Conclusion

Many older people have multiple problems caused by ageing and it can be difficult to uncover which problem is producing which particular symptom. It is important to identify which problems are related to normal ageing and those that are due to underlying physical and cognitive problems.

Several problems that arise from normal and abnormal ageing can be minimised by paying attention to practical issues. This book's emphasis is on the reduction of problems by altering techniques, providing assistive devices and ensuring that the environment facilitates not hinders full participation by residents.

Key points

- Ageing is a natural process that can add value to people's skills, but it can be accompanied by a propensity to experience physical and cognitive problems.
- Confusional states can arise from short-term treatable medical problems.
- Dementia is a clinical syndrome encompassing progressive impairments.
- Keeping active has benefits for both physical and cognitive function.

PART 2

Barriers

Barriers

CHAPTER 3

Removing barriers

Society, despite the introduction of the Disability Discrimination Act (DDA) 1995 Part III, continues to impose restrictions on people with access difficulties, causing barriers that prevent their full participation in society. Good inclusive design practices should not be confined to the interior of buildings. The exterior of care homes and the surrounding vicinity can either encourage or prohibit community involvement.

Barriers

The Department of Health's (2003a) report, 'Independence Matters: An Overview of the Performance of Social Care Services for Physically and Sensory Disabled People', outlines the social model of disability. It makes the important distinction between impairment and disability: 'Disability is shown as being caused by barriers or elements of social organisation that take little or no account of people who have impairments. Society disables people who have impairments because the way it has been set up prevents disabled people taking part in everyday life'. This report emphasises that to enable disabled people to play a full part in mainstream society, attention needs to be paid to the ways in which things are organised and structured to allow full participation.

Removing the barriers that exclude disabled people who have impairments can bring about this change. Barriers are not only physical in form, but include prejudice, stereotypes, inflexible organisational procedures and practices and inaccessible information, buildings and transport (Department of Health, 2003a).

A different perspective

Finkelstein's (1992) tale described a fictitious village specially designed for wheelchair users. This village was built on the outskirts of a town. It contained tracks for wheelchairs and buildings, with low doorways and lowered ceilings. After a flood, some able-bodied survivors from the original town sought refuge in the wheelchair users' village, but had difficulty adapting. They constantly walked into doorframes, and developed backache from bending over to negotiate their new environment. They twisted their legs and fell over in the wheelchair tracks. The caring, wheelchair-using medical profession recommended that the able-bodied should use a wheelchair permanently for health and social acceptability. 'The village doctors... recommended either a harness to keep the able-bodied bent double at wheelchair height or padded guards which were strapped to the forehead.'

This sardonic tale demonstrates how environments can handicap individuals. Access is not just about physically entering or leaving a building, important though that may be. It is, in essence, about social inclusion and the value society places on individuals.

Society creates barriers to participation, and as such, most can be removed or not made in the first place, just by adopting an attitude of open access for all. A generalist approach not only benefits those typically construed as disabled, such as wheelchair users or ambulant disabled people. There are physical barriers that prevent disabled people from real and meaningful participation in all of its forms, but there are wider manifestations of access problems in society. There are spin-off advantages for all. Struggling with access issues is equally a problem encountered by parents with prams or when accompanying young children.

What does the law say?

The Disability Discrimination Act (1995) was strengthened on 1 October 2004, requiring businesses and other organisations to take reasonable steps to tackle physical features that act as a barrier to disabled people who want to access their services. Providers of services to the general public now have to make 'reasonable adjustment to overcome physical barriers'. For example, if the main entrance cannot be adapted, an alternative side entrance is required. Proprietors must provide an 'access statement' if buildings are unable to comply with the building regulations, explaining why and describing alternative arrangements; for example, providing a bell or intercom to call an employee to attend to the disabled person. The DDA defines disability as '... a physical or mental impairment which has a substantial and long-term adverse effect on a person's ability to carry out normal day-to-day activities'.

Disability therefore extends to:

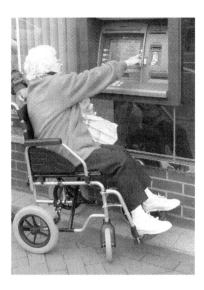

Cash machines: access can be difficult (© NRC 2004).

- Physical problems affecting range of movement, power, control or sensation
- Sensory impairments (deafness, visual problems and dual sensory impairments)
- Impairment of mental function (such as perceptual problems, cognitive problems and learning disabilities)
- Hidden disabilities where problems are not immediately apparent (such as heart disease, breathing problems, diabetes, epilepsy and dyslexia)

The legal position makes wide-ranging requirements on providers of services, focusing on access for all as a key principle, rather than meeting specific problems.

A new Disability Discrimination Act (2005) amends or extends existing provisions in the DDA 1995, including:

- making it unlawful for operators of transport vehicles to discriminate against disabled people
- making it easier for disabled people to rent property and for tenants to make disability-related adaptations
- making sure that private clubs with 25 or more members cannot keep disabled people out just because they have a disability
- extending protection to cover people who have HIV, cancer and multiple sclerosis from the moment they are diagnosed
- ensuring that discrimination law covers all the activities of the public sector
- requiring public bodies to promote equality of opportunity for disabled people

Universal inclusive design

Goldsmith's (1976) original publication *Designing for the Disabled* focused on the needs of disabled people. He later wrote *Universal Design* (Goldsmith, 2002), which encouraged architects, planners and occupational therapists to look beyond the prescribed minimum design standards by extending the parameters of normal provision.

If accessible buildings and easy-to-use items were designed from the start, fewer adaptations would be required. *Access to and Use of Buildings* (Office of the Deputy Prime Minister (ODPM) (2006) provides a blueprint for architects based on normative anthropometric data (the 'average person'). This document took effect on 1 May 2004, and dealt with the requirements of Part M of Schedule 1 to the Building Regulations Act 2000. Part M states that reasonable provision should be made for people to gain access to and use the building and its facilities.

Design considerations include the following:

- A new built house must have one entrance accessible by a wheelchair user.
- If a gradient is present, this should be minimal (less than 1:20).
- Revolving doors are no longer recommended in public buildings.
- The opening force at the lead edge of a door should be no greater than 20 N (newton force).

Barriers still exist

Although Goldsmith (1976, 2002) and many others presented a comprehensive case for an inclusive approach to access, there is still a long way to go. Many access problems can still be seen, for example:

- Lifts involving backward egress without a mirror on the wall to facilitate manoeuvring, instead of allowing forward access and egress.
- Heavy, difficult-to-open doors – although an increasing number of buildings, for example banks, have push-button assisted door openings.
- Narrow door widths and passages that prohibit passage.
- Solid doors with no visibility panels.
- Washbasins with difficult-to-turn taps, rather than one-action lever taps or sensor-operated taps.

- Loose stone covering to driveways, car parks and paths rather than tarmac, brick or concrete.
- Toilets designed for wheelchair users without mirrors that appear to assume that 'disabled' people are not concerned about their appearance.

Perhaps the term 'accessible' toilets should be used instead of 'disabled' toilets. This starts from the assumption that you want everybody to use the facilities – the young and the old, men and women, the tall and the short, the mobile and those with disabilities, those with child carriers and those with wheelchairs or walking frames. If creative thought is applied, accessibility issues can be solved with relatively little cost.

Progress made to date

The Disability Rights Commission (2003) produced several booklets, including *2004 – What it Means to You: a Guide for Service Providers*, which contains useful information on access issues. The DRC's goal of having a 'society where disabled people can participate fully as equal citizens' is gradually being achieved through the following examples:

- Levelling or ramping and widening entrances to shops.
- Wheelchair-accessible telephone booths and cash machines, although several do not permit sideways access to facilitate operation.
- Contrasting décor and tactile markings with visibility panels to help the safe mobility of visually impaired people.

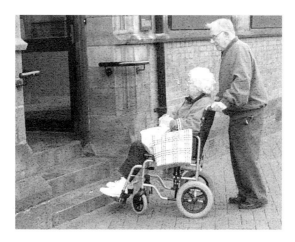

Not all buildings are accessible (© Julie Swann 2007).

- Practical help to negotiate transportation systems with raised kerbs at bus stops and buses that lower to facilitate access.
- Signage with large print and raised lettering and 'loop' systems.
- Paths with lower gradients (less than 1:20) with passing or resting places and accessible country paths without stiles.
- Pedestrian crossings that 'bleep' when it is safe to cross. Visually impaired people cannot locate the crossing easily, unlike in Berlin and Amsterdam, where crossings permanently give out an audible 'tick-tock' that quickens when it is safe to cross.
- Designing shops with plenty of seating and wide passageways and no internal steps unless a lift is available.
- Ramps as well as step access with suitable handrails.
- Free loan of scooters or wheelchairs, and supermarket trolleys that can be clipped onto a wheelchair or that have a high base to avoid bending.

Access when outside of the home

By sensible environmental planning and appropriate design strategies, 'disabled' people can participate more fully in a real and meaningful way.

- **Access into buildings**
Vehicles can be parked near the entrance, particularly in inclement weather. There is a new growing web site at `http://www.yourlevelbest.com/` with details of accessible venues, pubs and shops in the UK.

- **Access into toilets**
Sometimes access to the toilet area may be adequate, but if a toilet door opens inwards, this restricts the space. In a small cubicle, it is difficult to close the door for an average sized adult; for people with children, shopping bags or luggage, this often requires the occupant to move to the side of the toilet to close and open the doors. People using walking aids or a wheelchair and those who need assistance may not be able to gain access without leaving the door open. This can be a very humiliating experience. With foresight, most cubicles could easily have been made longer. Often, there is sufficient room to re-hang the door or make the cubicle space larger, as outward-opening doors provide greater access in an emergency, for example if a person has had a fall in the cubicle.

The Building Regulations – Part M (ODPM, 2006) recognise that 'the provision of an enlarged cubicle in a separate-sex toilet washroom can be of benefit to ambulant disabled people, as well as parents with children, and people (e.g. those with luggage) who need an enlarged space'.

For many people with mobility difficulties, accessing and using toilets away from home can be a stressful and difficult experience. Fortunately, most towns have an accessible toilet that is operated by a key obtained from the Royal Association for Disability and Rehabilitation (RADAR) tourist offices and some local authorities. The whereabouts of all National Key Scheme (NKS) toilets are listed in RADAR's (2005) *NKS Guide*, a useful publication to help locate accessible toilets for trips out with residents.

■ **Access in shops**
Several shops have level entrances and automatic door openings. Some have lifts and short ramps if there is a series of steps. A few shops have changing rooms for disabled customers with, for example, doors that open outwards to permit ease of access and door closure; a seat with armrests; adequate space and turning room within the cubicle for wheelchair access; a walking appliance; and an attendant.

Ensuring access is easy

Many physical problems are acquired throughout life. Reid (2004) states there are around 9.8 million adults and children in the UK affected by a disability. Anyone can become a 'disabled' person from injury, illness or ageing, causing problems that affect capacity to deal with daily life. Many people experience difficulties managing several flights of steps, even with a handrail. Ageing causes vision to deteriorate, a loss of dexterity and weakening of musculature. Loss of dexterity and deteriorating cognitive abilities hinder adapting to and managing new technology.

Conclusion

Access issues in the broadest sense are not just for 'disabled' people, but make life easier for everybody. The principles of inclusive design can be applied to a care home setting, and the next chapter discusses this concept.

Key points

- Society disables people by creating obstacles.
- Barriers prevent full participation and social inclusion.
- Good design that focuses on access for all helps minimise disability.

CHAPTER 4

Making care homes more accessible

Accessing buildings and services is not just about wheelchair users or people who have a limitation of mobility. The issues need to be looked at from a broad perspective: care homes can improve residents' lives and maintain levels of independence by adopting a positive approach to the subject. Consider, for example, the following problems:

- Impairment of hand function, causing limitation of movement, weak grip or loss of dexterity (perhaps resulting from arthritis, Parkinsonism, stroke or amputation) and resulting in problems with manipulating small items such as light switches, doorbells and door handles.
- Shortness of breath owing to chest or heart problems, leading to inability to walk long distances without frequent rests.
- Cognitive or sensory impairments, producing difficulty finding way around and problems locating and reading signage.

None of these problems requires the provision of ramps or wider doorways, yet all of them can be handicapping if an environment imposes barriers that prevent full participation.

Care standards: implications for care homes

On 1 April 2004, the Commission for Social Care Inspection (CSCI) acquired responsibility for the inspection of all care homes. CSCI regulates social care services in accordance with statutory regulations and the National Minimum Standards issued by the Department of Health (2003b). The 2003 National Minimum Standards stemmed from the Care Standards Act (2000), providing a benchmark for care homes. The scale below is used to indicate the extent to which standards have or have not been met:

4 = Standard exceeded (commendable)
3 = Standard met (no shortfalls)

2 = Standard almost met (minor shortfalls)
1 = Standard not met (major shortfalls)
0 = Not assessed or was not applicable on this occasion

CSCI inspectorate reports

At present, care homes have a yearly 'announced' inspection, for which they can prepare. At this inspection, all relevant National Minimum Standards should be reviewed. Care homes also have a yearly 'unannounced' inspection. Unannounced or complaints investigation inspection reports may not review all of the National Minimum Standards, but may focus on specific service areas. CSCI inspection reports are obtainable from: http://www.csci.org. uk/RegisteredServicesDirectory/rsquicksearch.asp.

The Department of Health (2003b) states that all care homes should comply with the National Minimum Care Home Regulations. These standards specify door entrance widths and minimum space within a room.

■ **Entrance to the room**
Standard 22.5 states that:

> Doorways into communal areas, service users' rooms, bathing and toilet facilities and other spaces to which wheelchair users have access, should be of width sufficient to allow wheelchair users adequate access. In all newly built homes, new extensions to homes and first time registrations doorways into areas to which wheelchair users have access should have a clear opening of 800 mm.

■ **Space and contents of a room**
Standard 34 provides a basic list of furniture. Standard 23 states that room sizes of 12 m² should be provided for wheelchairs users and that 10 m² will suffice for other single users in existing homes. However, this fails to allow for the fact that some wheeled walking frames will require almost as much turning space and take up as much floor space as a wheelchair user. Neither does this cater for the furniture belonging to a resident, and therefore problems may arise with access within the room.

It is important that all staff familiarise themselves with all of the standards. Although the standards emphasise the importance of access for ambulant disabled and wheelchair users, they pay insufficient attention to many of the physical problems experienced by people who have or problems affecting upper limbs, sensation or cognition.

Table 4.1 National minimum care standards: standard 22.

22.1	The registered person demonstrates that an assessment of the premises and facilities has been made by suitably qualified persons, including a qualified occupational therapist, with specialist knowledge of the client groups catered for, and provides evidence that the recommended disability equipment has been secured or provided and environmental adaptations made to meet the needs of service users.
22.2	Service users have access to all parts of service users' communal and private space, through the provision of ramps and passenger lifts, where required to achieve this.
22.3	The home provides grab rails and other aids in corridors, bathrooms, toilets, communal rooms and where necessary, in service users' own accommodation.
22.4	Aids, hoists and assisted toilets and baths are installed that are capable of meeting the assessed needs of service users.
22.5	Doorways into communal areas, service users' rooms, bathing and toilet facilities and other spaces to which wheelchair users have access have a clear opening width of 800 mm.
22.6	Facilities, including communication aids (e.g. a loop system) and signs are provided to assist the needs of all service users, taking account of the needs, for example, of those with hearing impairment, visual impairment, dual sensory impairments, learning disabilities or dementia or other cognitive impairment, where necessary.
22.7	Storage areas are provided for aids and equipment, including wheelchairs.
22.8	Call systems with an accessible alarm facility are provided in every room.

Inspecting for better lives: proposed CSCI changes

CSCI (2005) produced a document titled *Inspecting for Better Lives – Delivering change*. This document contains proposed CSCI modernisation plans, and is available electronically from http://www.csci.org.uk/PDF/ibl_2.pdf. Most future inspections will be unannounced and include a risk assessment of how the service affects its users. This CSCI document mentions '... we will start to ask people who use care services to act as "mystery shoppers" to find out what's happening on a day-to-day basis...'. It also states that, 'Self-assessment of services will be accepted and all providers will take responsibility for improving their services'.

Access issues within the care environment

Any design of a care home, or even a small extension, should be inclusive in design to facilitate access and safety. This will save expensive future altera- tions. The physical layout of care homes should also provide an environment to allow the resident to function at their highest level possible. Before a CSCI inspectorate visit, Crisp (2004) suggests that staff should make 'observational tours', specifically looking at the accessibility of equipment for residents and access to and around the building. Some obvious adaptations and assistive devices are mentioned in standard 22 (Table 4.1), such as ramps, passenger lifts and grab rails. CSCI recommend that access audits are carried out and some independent occupational therapists provide this service.

When looking at access issues in a care home, it is useful to make several journeys with various problems in mind. As a general rule, it is helpful to go through the home checking each room with a mindset of what it might be like for the particular resident, bearing in mind their physical and cognitive prob- lems. Trying to 'step into someone's shoes' can help increase understanding of how a home's environment may restrict residents' abilities further. Imagine being a new resident: look for features that will enhance access or make life difficult, and therefore need attention.

Another method of understanding problem areas is to accompany residents on their journey around the home. Allow residents to open doors or turn lights on for themselves. Strategic placement of essential items can make the differ- ence between a resident doing an activity independently and requiring help. It is important to adapt designs to residents' needs and to look at residents' anthropometrics. For example: an individual's range of movement, coordina- tion and strength will affect the position of handrails.

Sources of information

Many books and guidelines provide details of recommended heights for gen- eral use (Goldsmith, 1976, 2002). Examples of good design features, heights of rails and ramps, toilets and room layouts are provided in the 'Building Reg- ulations' (ODPM, 2006).

Access issues and audits

When care homes are built or refurbished, the emphasis may be placed on physical access and a resident's hidden handicaps may inadvertently be overlooked. Examples of hidden handicaps include breathing difficulties, heart problems and sensory or perceptual problems. It is important to ensure that access is provided at all times to facilities so that residents can use them. Table 4.2 contains a list of some common minor issues that may need addressing. Several items can be addressed and resolved by 'good housekeeping', for example:

- One residential home had a public telephone in a quiet area of the home but access was blocked as the area was used for wheelchair storage.
- Emergency pull-cords or their handles are often broken or not within reach of a resident. These should be checked regularly as a cracked or broken handle can easily damage ageing fragile skin.

Environmental obstacles

With some slight adaptations, rooms in care homes can be altered to make allowance for any impairment that a resident may have. If physical obstacles are minimised, there will be less need for equipment. For example, if single-action lever taps are provided to washbasins as a standard item, no tap turners or conversion to lever taps will be required. Table 4.3 illustrates some common problems and suggests the type of changes to the environment that can be made to minimise problems for residents.

How to make the environment easier to cope with

Many homes have an ageing population and some residents may have major cognitive deficits due to dementia. The environment may require additional modification to help them understand their environment and to compensate for cognitive deterioration in addition to modifications relating to physical access. The consensus on principles of design is that environments should (Marshall, 2001):

- 'compensate for disability;
- maximise independence;

Table 4.2 Areas to consider when doing an access audit.

Outdoors

Is there a designated disabled-parking space or room to alight near the front or rear entrance?

Is seating provided near the front entrance for those with a limited standing ability?

Can the doorbell be reached from a wheelchair and is it easy to locate?

Is there a covered area by the entrance?

Indoors – communal areas

Do automatic doors stay open long enough to permit safe passage?

Is there sufficient signage to aide orientation?

Is there seating midway from the lounge area to the dining room, toilet and bedrooms for residents who have breathing problems or tire easily?

Is there contrasting ribbed flooring in front of lifts and at the top and bottom of the staircase to aid visually impaired people?

Have handrails been installed at both sides of staircases and do they extend 300 mm beyond the end of the staircase?

Are handrails provided on both sides of ramps?

Are alarm pull-cords 100 mm above the floor and reachable?

Indoors – individual rooms

Can your resident open the door to the room?

Are the alarm cords within easy reach of the bed and chair?

Can your resident turn on light switches and manage the bedside light?

Is the furniture, including drawer units and wardrobes, easy to open?

Can residents dial and hold a phone?

Is the lighting sufficient within the communal areas?

Indoors – ensuite rooms

Is the alarm cord within reach when the resident is on the toilet?

Have handrails been provided in ensuite bathrooms?

Can the resident operate the taps?

Is the toilet paper dispenser within reach?

Can the resident manage to extract paper or is a single leaf dispenser needed?

Table 4.3 Some solutions to common problems.

External to the room	Suggested solution
Identifying the door	Different coloured bedroom doors that contrast visually with surroundings Use large numbers or a picture on the door to generate appropriate signage Ensure the level of lighting is sufficient and replace single bulbs with multiple light bulb fittings in case one 'blows'
Using a key, if the door is lockable	Key turners can help if hand function is poor, or change type of locking mechanism
Opening the door	Replace doorknobs with lever handles
Managing steps at the entrance to the room	A risk assessment must be carried out. Handrails at either side of the door may be needed to help steady the resident

Within the room	Suggested solution
Opening the door	Replace doorknobs with lever handles
Locking a door from the inside	Latch-type of bolt that can be opened by staff from the outside in an emergency
Closing the door easily	Wheelchair users can be helped by the provision of a horizontal grab rail on the inside of the door
Reaching the alarm pull cord	Lengthen pull-cords and use extension leads on push-button from bed and chair assistance call pads
Operating bedside lamp	Touch (sensor) lamp
Reach and operate telephone	Large buttons for ease of use Speaker telephone or cordless phone system
Manage curtains	Pull-cord system
Open and reach drawers	Place essential items within reach. Replace door furniture with larger knob or D-shaped handle. Place knob/handle in middle of draw if resident only has the use of one hand
Reach personal items and toiletries	Place everyday items within reach
Manage taps	Single-action lever taps or fit a lever tap conversion kit
Reach toilet paper and extract	Place paper within reach. Consider interleaved toilet paper or a toilet roll that 'locks' each turn

Table 4.3 (*continued*)

Within the room (*continued*)	Suggested solution
Height of mirror	Provide a lower sited mirror for a wheelchair user or a full-length mirror with shatterproof glass
Towel holder within reach	Reposition so that it is reachable from the sink and from a seated position
Height of electric sockets within reach	Raise the position of the socket
Position of sockets within reach	Reposition furniture to give access to sockets
Personal safe within room	Is it reachable and easy to operate?

- enhance self-esteem and confidence;
- demonstrate care for staff;
- be orientating and understandable;
- reinforce personal identity;
- welcome relatives and the local community;
- allow control of stimuli'.

Some care homes are specifically designed to cope with a population of confused elderly people. The layout of these homes makes orientation, way finding and daily living activities easier, not more difficult; for example:

- **Layout of the home**
  - All corridors lead to somewhere safe, e.g. and enclosed garden area, a reception area or a small setting area, instead of corridors leading to a fire door that residents may want to escape though.
  - An enclosed garden area with interesting safe features, e.g. bubble fountain, sculpture, gazebo and several exits from the home so that wanderers can walk safely (outdoor wandering spaces), instead of locked external doors.
  - Subtly placed assistive equipment to help compensate for problems, e.g. rails and non-slip floors.
  - Features to differentiate areas, corridors and floors, e.g. using plants, large pictures or scenes painted on the wall.

- **Decoration**
  - Corridors decorated in different colour themes or with contrasting borders to aid orientation rather than painted/decorated the same.
  - Interior design using non-institutional, strong yet calming colours of blue, pink, lemon or lilac instead of magnolia. Pale colours may be hard to see, but very bright colours can be over stimulating.
  - Contrasting colours to help differentiate where the floor finishes and the wall starts; conversely, exits or 'prohibited' rooms can be camouflaged by painting doors the same colour as the walls.
- **Signage**
  - Clear signage of floor number or strong wall colour opposite lift e.g. blue floor, green floor, pink floor to help to identify the floor a resident has reached.
- **Communal rooms**
  - Clearly defined sections within a large room or small rooms that are familiar and homely in style with different functions.
  - A focal point in a room, e.g. a fireplace, a bookcase or a display cabinet rather than just chairs and tables placed around a room, with ambient lighting to give a cosy effect.
  - Homely touches like cushions, pictures and ornaments, perhaps in a toughened glass cabinet, in place of institutionalised décor.
  - Provision of props for interaction and stimulation, e.g. cards, dominoes and magazines, sited within reach.
  - Replace a custodial environment with a normalising environment that allows past activities to be carried on, e.g. making a cold drink, pegging washing on the line, pottering in a garden shed.
  - Have a chest of drawers in a room that is full of items for people to rummage though and tidy, e.g. paper, balls of wool, magazines, tea towels and clothes pegs.
  - Arrange chairs and dining tables in social groups to encourage social interaction (sociopetal), not ones that discourage social interaction (sociofugal).
- **Toilets**
  - Install a contrasting coloured toilet seat and put coloured disinfectant blocks in the cistern to assist identification.
  - Remove the waste paper baskets or any similar items in the toilet if they are mistaken for a toilet.
  - Sufficient lighting in the hall leading to the toilet and passive infrared (PIR) lighting that comes on when passing the toilet or as soon as the toilet door opens.
  - Consider providing a urinal, as these are often easier for male residents to manage.

■ **Bedrooms**
  - Large enough for personal furniture to be brought into the home.
  - Use two different contrasting coloured sheets to help the resident find the way into bed and turn back the top sheet.
  - Provide a sensor light or PIR light that activates when the resident gets out of bed.
  - Ensure the room is in darkness and use 'black out material' to discourage residents from getting out of bed.
  - Consider using plug-in 'nightlights' or soft lighting to minimise disorientation if residents wake up and wander during the night.
  - Use external aids (Burns, 2005) such as non-electric memory aids, diaries, calendars, wipe clean boards, notice boards and memo recorders.

■ **General safety aspects**
  - Unobtrusive safety devices, e.g. staff call buttons hidden from view.
  - Alarm systems including pressure pads adjacent beds to monitor night-time wanderers.
  - Remove and lock away toxic cleaning products for safety.

■ **Lighting**
  - Sensor lights beside bed and PIR lighting in corridors to illuminate areas of low lighting, as inadequate levels of lighting increase the risk of falling.
  - Leave ordinary lights on in the main rooms and external areas. Sensor lights (PIR) in the house and gardens are useful, but some residents may find them disturbing.
  - Good task lighting in areas like lifts, entrances to doors etc.

Some of the above are little touches that cost very little and can be incorporated into refurbishing redecorating schemes. They will make the environment easier to manage, providing a more sociable setting and helping to remove any environmental factors that can trigger maladaptive behaviour. In bedroom and ensuite areas it is particularly important to make changes slowly and in ways that will support the resident, and to remember that as the person's dementia progresses their abilities and capacities to cope will change. In addition to ensuring that access and features cope with physical problems, it is important to consider the sensory and cognitive abilities of residents.

Looking at behaviour

In tandem with looking at the environment, it is important to look at the ABC (antecedent, behaviour itself and the consequence) of a resident's behaviour. It is often the way that behaviour is dealt with (the consequence) that can escalate or minimise a negative behaviour patterns. Finding the cause of maladaptive behaviour can reduce or remove the behaviour. Review sessions or staff meetings can be used to explore problem areas and to find simple and cost-effective solutions. It is important to address areas that can retain a resident's level of abilities and independence for as long as possible, whilst making access easier.

Conclusion

If the environment is adapted to cope with an ageing population this will make mobility and living in a care home more easier for the resident and prolong their level of independence and provide a more socially interactive place to live. When alterations are carried out to premises, it makes sense to make sure that the positions of items like lighting, switches or door handles are accessible for most people. With a little thought, life can be made easier for the residents and they can maintain and improve their level of independence.

Environmental factors can hinder cognitive abilities or help them. Making a resident's environment more accessible need not involve costly adaptations to property; often, simple solutions and good housekeeping issues involving minor changes can make life easier.

Key points

- Homes should be viewed from the perspective of the resident.
- Ensure access is maintained by 'good housekeeping'.
- Assess for and provide assistive devices to maintain residents' independence.
- Understand the impact of hidden disabilities by looking beyond obvious physical or cognitive dysfunction.

CHAPTER 5

Turning gardens into multi-sensory experiences

First impressions often count, and the first view that potential residents, their family, friends or the person that is responsible for assisting them to find a care home have is of the exterior of a home. Although not every care home can be sited in acres of land, even a small courtyard area can be transformed into an attractive feature, viewable all year round.

Although gardening is construed as an active hobby, all can enjoy the pleasures of a being in or surrounded by a garden. Gardens can provide active or passive enjoyment. They can be places to reflect, to reminisce, to contemplate or to simply to look out onto. A garden should be an integral, interesting part of a care home environment, no matter how small the area available. With forward planning, gardens can be designed to provide enjoyment and a safe outdoor environment to stimulate all senses.

Today, we are far more aware of the physical difficulties that prevent full enjoyment of a garden. To enable people of all ages and abilities to participate and to enjoy basic facilities without the need for adaptations, the concept of inclusive design should extend into outdoor spaces.

Redesigning a garden

There are many books and articles on designing gardens for wheelchair users, ambulant disabled persons and visually impaired gardeners. The ideas can be applied to ensure inclusive design with a care home. Some features that aid access are provided in Table 5.1. Seating areas grouped together, with spaces for wheelchair users, can encourage social interaction. Ask several staff and residents to journey through the garden, pinpointing areas of sensory stimulation or relaxation, to plan appropriate seating areas.

Table 5.1 Designing an inclusive garden (refer to *Building Regulations* (2000) for dimensions).

- **Entrances and exits**
  - No thresholds at entrances or exits to garden.
  - Large external and internal mats to wipe feet and clean wheels/ walking aids on.

- **Paths and surfaces**
  - Pathways wide enough to permit passage by a wheelchair and ambulant disabled person with an attendant or provision of 'passing places'.
  - Straight paths with focal features to aid orientation of residents with visual impairments, e.g. sculpture and water features that emit sound.
  - Concrete or brick edges to prevent wheelchair tipping over the edge.
  - Gradients of less than 1:10.
  - Handrails adjacent to any steps or paths.
  - Even surfaces that are easy to manoeuvre over and anti-slip.
  - Hard landscaping rather than a lawn area, using decking or large slabs particularly when access is needed.

- **Seating**
  - Abundance of resting places set back from a path (avoids being a trip hazard).
  - Seating by focal points in the sun and the shade, e.g. bubble fountains, bird tables, sensory gardens, under trees.
  - Tables with spaces to park a wheelchair alongside and knee access so a resident can use the table.

- **Raised planting**
  - Raised beds can be made of brick, concrete or treated wood (e.g. railway sleepers) and should provide access for wheelchair users.
  - Hanging baskets and sturdy flowerpots can add interest to areas of a garden or path.
  - Avoid plants that are harmful if touched or ingested.

- **Lighting**
  - Up-lighters can enhance gardens on a dull winter evening.
  - Lighting can aid visual guidance.

- **Wildlife**
  - Birdfeeders, waterfalls and shallow ponds all attract wildlife.

Sources of information

Libraries have many books on designing or redesigning any type or size of garden. Books on gardening for busy people can provide a wealth of ideas to be used in care homes. Pavey (1999) helps the reader to create an 'outside room' that is 'a place of relaxation – a bolt-hole from the pressures that life throws at us all'. He describes redesigning a garden in stages, particularly if there are budget constraints.

Many care homes prefer simple, attractive, low-maintenance gardens. Local gardening clubs or colleges that run gardening courses may be interested in a 'live project' to help you redesign a garden area. Cowley (2004) describes how, in 2002, BUPA approached Thrive, a national disability and gardening charity, to help create sensory gardens enlisting the help of volunteers and community groups.

TV programmes such as *Ground Force* and *Garden Fronts* provide inspiration for low-maintenance gardens and gardens designed for a wheelchair user. There is a sample of a low-maintenance wheelchair-friendly garden online at http://www.bbc.co.uk/gardening/design/des_ins/leaf_pages/23.shtml. The BBC (2006) web site contains a free download of *Virtual Garden*, which takes the user though designing to creating a garden in two-dimensional and three-dimensional formats. Different forms of seating, fencing, planting and ground cover can be experimented with, although there is limited choice of features and foliage.

Themed gardens

Themes can be used, for example English tea garden, Mediterranean garden, Japanese garden, herb garden, nature garden or a courtyard design surrounding a patio area. Plants grown in containers add interest to a bare wall, although ideally they should be planted in the ground. Chalfont (2005) provides a visual template for a garden within a dementia care setting, encouraging users to venture outside 'just to see what is going on', suggesting that gardening spaces should relate to each other so that 'people can observe the action, comment on it and develop a desire to participate'.

Providing a year-round garden

Visual impact is important, and ideally gardens should be pleasant and view-able from inside the year through. This is particularly important in a care home

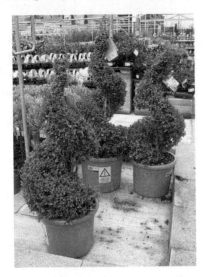 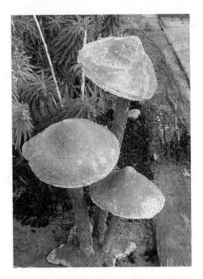

All year-round sculptural features (© NRC 2006 (left) and Julie Swann 2007 (right).

setting, when some residents may not venture outside. Conservatories and strategic lighting will extend the hours that a garden can be enjoyed. Stebbings' (2005) book lists over 500 plants and thousands of companions that help create an attractive garden throughout the seasons. It provides planting combinations and a useful cross-referenced profile of plants; such as identifying which season they are in bud, flower or leaf.

> Rather than be defeated by the changing seasons, we should rejoice in the variety that they bring and make the most of each time of the year (Stebbings, 2005).

Sensory gardens

Sensory gardens encourage exploration and interaction with objects; therefore beds should be small and approachable on several sides to facilitate access. Sensory gardens can target one sense – for example, a fragrant garden – or have several separate sections aimed at specific senses, or the whole area can be multi-sensory. Although sensory gardens specifically aim to stimulate all of the senses of sight, smell, touch, hearing and taste, some sensory stimulation is inherent in all gardens.

■ Visual stimulation

English gardens are very colourful in spring, summer and autumn. Plants full of nectar attract butterflies and pollinating insects. In late autumn, winter and early spring there is little colour apart from evergreen shrubs and trees. Therefore, rather than focusing on colours, incorporate plants that have unusual shapes. 'Architectural' plants will provide an interesting view all year round. Shaw (2005) describes an architectural plant as having 'a strong shape, an exotic appearance, an evergreen presence or an unusual quality that can visually improve its surroundings'. Her book is full of ideas for conservatory and outdoor planting, including sections on palms, ferns, grasses, climbers and trees with unusual bark colours and shapes.

Small sculptures, wooden structures and water features will add interest, for example pagodas, arches, gazebos and bubble fountains. A simple Zen garden can be made of three large rocks on a bed of stone with a dry slate stream. Plant, bark and leaf colours can complement or perhaps contrast against the surrounding walls, screens or fences. Bird feeders will encourage birds into the garden and can be placed at wheelchair height to allow access by a wheelchair user.

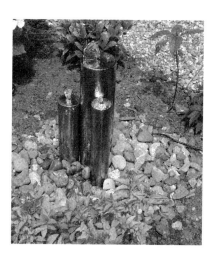

A safe water feature (© NRC 2006).

■ Olfactory stimulation

Scented plants, such as the curry plant, evening primrose, honeysuckle, lilac, lily-of-the-valley, mock orange, roses, night-scented stock, sweet peas and wisteria, fragrance the air without the need to touch. Many smells, including subtle fragrances such as daffodil and violets, evoke memories of bygone days. Sunny areas allow the more fragrant flowers to grow. Herb sections, such as

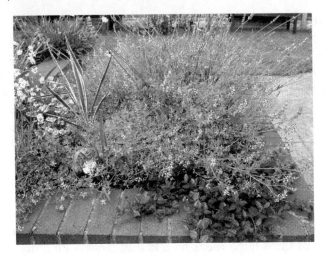

Raised bed: full of textures and aromas (© Julie Swann 2007).

thyme, fennel, mint and rosemary, add fragrance and are useful in home cooking. Scent arises from other sources, for example during a barbeque, when logs, charcoal, herbs and food are added. Lavender, lemon balm and other scents/oils enhance cognitive ability and can be relaxing, soothing or stimulating. Aromatherapy oils and scented candles will blend with the more natural smells of cut grass and add to visual impact.

■ Tactile stimulation

Many plants are wonderful to touch, with silky or fragranced leaves activated by brushing against them or by slightly crushing – for example, coriander, lemon balm, mint and scented geranium. Tactile plants can be placed in pots near a path. Different surfaces can be used for raised beds and concrete containers can be made more interesting with a pebble top or the edges brushed with yoghurt to encourage moss growth. Residents may enjoy cutting flowers or arranging them. Plants can be dried and used in craft activities.

■ Auditory stimulation

Auditory stimulation can be provided by natural or activated sounds. Natural sounds arise from birds, wildlife or rainwater trickling down into a container that will attract the birds to drink and bathe. Plants and trees provide rustling sounds in the path of a breeze. Activated sounds include wind chimes attached above arches to created gentle noises and water features, such as a mini-waterfall, water urn or bubble fountain with a flow of water.

- **Taste**

Tabor (2002) provides chapters on identifying herbs that are visually effective, useful for the kitchen, provide fragrance and can be used in crafts or just for cut flowers. Edible produce, such as strawberries and tomatoes, can be grown outside of doorways or in the greenhouse.

- **Other senses**

Additional to the main five senses, there are many more sensory pathways that can be stimulated in a garden. We perceive changes in temperature and gardens should provide areas of sun and shade, essential if residents have sensitive skin or are sensitive to heat. Several web sites contain lists of plants to stimulate various senses, such as Noahs (*sic*) Ark Wildlife Gardens (`http://www.noah-sarkgardens.co.uk/`), which states:

> A sensory garden is an area purposefully set out in separate beds that provide a wide range of sensory experiences in close proximity. Such an area provides a valuable site that can be used for relaxation, stimulation or even education, and a seating or rest area would normally be included in the design.

Dangerous plants

Thorny, prickly plants and weeds, like roses and brambles, can hurt if a fall occurs or limbs become entangled, but several garden plants, fruit and herbs can cause considerable harm if touched. As many herbs, fruit, flowers and vegetables can cause problems if ingested, it is safer to avoid plants that can cause harm if touched or eaten.

Care is required if there is a likelihood of a resident ingesting a poisonous plant, perhaps mistaking it for edible berries. It is important to realise that severe reactions in residents can arise. Monkshood is a very dangerous plant and all parts, particularly the root, are poisonous and fatal. Collins' (2001) useful book provides photographs of poisonous plants that 'have adverse effect on humans whether through contact or ingestion'. Tabor's (2002) chapter on useful herbs has a section on toxic herbs that identifies many side effects of the common herbs grown in many gardens for culinary purposes. Table 5.2 contains extracts from Collins' (2001) book that describes some of the most dangerous plants.

Table 5.2 Information on some of the most dangerous plants – extracted from Collins (2001).

Plant/fruit	Hazardous part	Symptoms
Delphinium and larkspur	Seeds and leaves if ingested	Sudden death; paralysis, difficulty breathing and weak irregular pulse
Foxglove	All. Contains digitalis, which affects the heart, causing sudden death	Ingestion causes vomiting and diarrhoea and small amounts affect the heart
Hellebore (Christmas Rose)	All parts	Delirium, convulsions and respiratory failure; death
Laurel	All, especially leaves (contain hydrocyanic acid) and kernels of fruit	Convulsions and respiratory distress
Lily of the valley	Whole plant	Cardio glycosides act on the heart, causing low, irregular pulse, severe abdominal pain, vomiting, dilated pupils. Clammy skin, delirium, coma and death
Lupin.	All parts especially the seeds.	Slows down the heart rate and respiratory system if ingested. Stomach pains, diarrhoea and vomiting.
Sweet pea	Seeds	Ingestion causes vomiting, diarrhoea and temporary muscle paralysis
Tobacco plant	Leaves contain nicotine. Very poisonous and easily absorbed into skin	Fatal if ingested
Celery and parsley	Sap if in contact with the sun in daylight	Irritation and blistering
Globe artichoke	Sap	Skin irritation and dermatitis
Rhubarb	Leaf blade contains oxalic acid. Stem is safe if removed 5 cm below leaf	Ingestion can cause muscle and kidney damage, coma and even death
Thyme	All. Oil is poisonous but small quantities may be safely used in cooking	Ranges from headache, dizziness, nausea, stomach pain, convulsions, cardiac and respiratory problems Soreness and inflammation from skin contact.
Tomato	Root, stem and leaves	Gastroenteritis, constipation, weakness and paralysis

Gardens as outdoor rooms

Gardens can be conceptualised as outdoor rooms and there are an increasing number of retail outlets that sell foliage and structural items. Several companies specialising in assistive equipment stock tools to enable disabled people to tend gardens more easily. Gardening equipment is explored in Chapter 19.

Involving other people

Residents can be involved in all aspects of gardening, even if a person is just watching someone sowing seeds. Later visits to the seedlings, as they grow, can assist in reality orientation and meaningful daily life. Ways of encouraging residents to participate actively in gardening are discussed in Chapter 19. Gardening can be a focal point of an active social community.

Conclusion

Gardens are places to 'sit and watch the world go by' or to enjoy actively. By planning a garden, enjoyment can be provided all year round to residents, staff and visitors and become an integral aspect of care.

Key points

- Gardens are integral parts of a care home and local community, providing beneficial interactions at all levels.
- Inclusive design ensures that all ages and levels of ability can enjoy a garden.
- Good garden design and architectural plants gives all-year-round pleasure.
- Sensory stimulation enhances a garden's therapeutic value.
- Care is needed to minimise the potential dangers of some plants.

Different approaches

CHAPTER 6

The importance of assessment

To 'assess', as defined in the *Cambridge Learner's Dictionary* (Cambridge University Press, 2003), is 'to judge or decide the amount, value, quality or importance of; to evaluate'. The Care Standards Act 2000 (Department of Health, 2000) defines assessment as the collection and interpretation of data. By adopting simple and basic principles of assessment, care home staff can improve their understanding of methods to promote an individual's social and health-care development.

When people enter care at times of crisis it is difficult to facilitate a smooth transition. There are, however, a number of steps that can be taken to ease the process and minimise the potential for deep-rooted psychological reactions. Transition into care is discussed in Chapter 1. Good understanding and assessment of residents' needs, when shared by all significant staff, ensure that effective coordinated care is provided to meet individual needs.

Continuous assessment

No single assessment document captures needs forever, as circumstances change and further needs develop over time. Assessment is not a 'one-off' event, but part of a continuum quantifying changes in a resident's function. With accurate assessment, interventions can be planned, goals established and appropriate referrals made to other service providers. A clear assessment procedure within a residential care environment is therefore essential.

Types of assessment

There are two main types of assessment, informal and formal.

■ Informal assessment
This is carried out on a day-to-day basis, often purely by observation. For example, when encountering a new situation or person, judgements are formed

quickly, in an automatic and subconscious way. Many people have 'gut feel-ings' when meeting someone for the first time. Considerable information can be obtained by observing appearance (clothing, posture, physique, facial expression and movement patterns), attitude and communication skills (words, tone, speed, non-verbal signals and body language). Many forms of perception help place facts and feelings into a framework, to enable decisions to be made that an individual believes to be correct at the time. However, first impressions are not always the most reliable, and a more systematic framework helps to minimise bias.

■ Formal assessment

This is a more structured approach. As assessment is open to inter-observer error, standardised testing helps reduce this by:

- Providing uniformity of procedure – all assessments are carried out in the same manner by assessors.
- Providing reliability – reduction of inter-observer error ensures that assessors will produce the same results and scores.
- Validity – measuring what it should measure.
- Providing scoring systems with normative data on the population so that results can be compared, for example, across age and gender.

Assessment within the care home setting

Assessment holistically considers both strengths and development areas within a social and physical context. Assessment processes need to recognise physical or mental frailty, yet view the individual in broader dimensions, as individuals are not defined by their physical or mental frailty. It is inappropriate to refer to someone as 'the person with MS in Room 22' or 'the demented person in Room 13'. People are complex beings living and functioning within a social setting. Care staff should identify and meet the unique and separate needs of individual residents. Most residents have the capacity for self-determination and staff should recognise the positive skills inherent with each individual. Much attention needs to be paid to the strengths and capacities of individuals to undertake tasks for themselves, as well as focusing on individual problems and difficulties.

The National Minimum Care Standards for Care Homes for Older People (Department of Health, 2002a) introduced several standards that directly relate to practical activities with residential care. Standards 12–15 of this Act deal with the social contact and activities of service users. There is an expectation on care homes to provide a varied and flexible routine of daily living and activities (Standard 12).

It is possible to use a number of different assessment tools that can be of value to comply with the care standards regulations. Inspectors look for evidence that care homes meet the assessed needs of service users and that changing needs continue to be met. Formal recording of assessment is therefore vital. Assessment is not only a formal requirement, but also a desirable activity in its own right.

Single assessment process

Many people report being passed from one agency to another and re-telling their tale to many different professionals. At times of vulnerability, this can be very frustrating and disempowering. The National Service Framework for Older People (Department of Health, 2001a) introduced the idea of a single assessment process (SAP) to avoid duplication of assessments and to ensure that older people receive appropriate, effective and timely responses to their health and social care needs, with professional resources used effectively. The development of the SAP intends to ensure that people who enter residential care will have an appropriate multidisciplinary assessment that is coordinated and holistic in its approach.

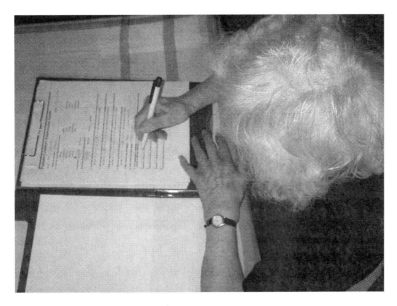

Self assessment (© Julie Swann 2007).

The Department of Health's (2004a) guidelines on the SAP provide advice on specific assessment scales that can be used in the assessment of older people's needs and circumstances under the SAP. The Department of Health (2002b) provided guidelines on suitable assessment criteria. Although aimed at local NHS bodies and local authorities, this contains useful material that care homes may find valuable. This document provided an overview of tests on specific areas, for example:

- Activities of daily living
- Mobility and balance
- Cognitive impairment and memory

It is impossible to guarantee that an assessment process will work well all the time, but a solid framework enables a better service to be provided and the choice taken to enter a residential setting becomes more likely to be a needs-driven and positive choice.

Start of assessment

The majority of individuals moving into a residential or nursing home environment will have had a community care assessment. This can involve health and social care staff. Interprofessional collaboration is essential. The care plan from the community care assessment forms the basis of a care home's assessment. It is important that internal systems and procedures are in place to translate the care plan into actual daily living. Assessment of residents by care staff occurs from first contact, perhaps by admission meetings or discussions with relevant people. All staff must know the procedures that the home adopts, with clear lines of responsibility and accountability for undertaking assessment.

Whatever assessment tools are used the assessment should include observation of, at least, the following:

- Physical and mental capabilities.
- Limitations owing to physical or cognitive problems.
- Methods of approaching tasks.
- Use of assistive equipment and adaptations.
- Ability to cope with the environment.

This information can be used to help plan appropriate care, as well as operating as a guide to determine suitable activities for residents. Care staff can use a separate resident's profile to record assessment and preferences to help in the planning of appropriate practical activities. Essential information on previous lifestyle, medical problems, medication, communication skills, physical abilities, functional abilities and interests need to be recorded. The family network, as well as any friends, neighbours, and other residents or relatives who have regular contact with the individual, should also be considered. Completing a resident's profile focuses on the abilities of a resident and methods that can be used to improve his or her quality of life. This alone can be motivating. By assessing a resident's level of function and abilities, strengths and problem areas are identified. Additionally, a baseline of function is established to compare function over a period of time and to assess improvement or deterioration in abilities.

The information within existing in-house assessments may provide sufficient detail, particularly if there is a section on recreational activities, hobbies or leisure – so 'why reinvent the wheel'? Alternatively, one of the many commercially available tests may be useful, or care homes may wish to compile their own. Whatever form of assessment and intervention is selected, records should be kept. This is useful for sharing with other members of staff who may not be on duty at that particular time, and demonstrates positive intervention.

Outcomes of assessment using a resident's profile

A resident's profile can identify desirable outcomes to enhance lifestyle, improve function and abilities, and perhaps achieve a greater degree of independence. Assessment may uncover areas of difficulty that need addressing and areas of ability that can be enhanced. Problem areas can cause difficulties with activities of daily living and recreation that small assistive devices can address. These problems are explored in other chapters.

Case study

- Resident A previously enjoyed bingo but his vision has deteriorated.
  - Large print bingo cards are available or can be made and an eyesight test arranged.
- Resident B has loss of arm function in one side (hemiparesis).
  - Some adapted cutlery and crockery facilitate eating.

Care staff may discover a common interest or a common problem area that can be concentrated on within a programme of activities, perhaps on a small group basis. Assessment may identify that referral is needed to outside agencies, such as the continence advisor, district nurse, physiotherapist or occupational therapist.

A regular review

Assessment is a continuous process, subject to adaptation and amendment. It is important that progress is reviewed regularly against set targets. This should include the residents and their carers. The review should be formally recorded with new targets established based upon clear and defined outcomes.

Conclusion

All care staff working within residential care should share the values and principles of maximising independence, respecting individuals and maximising self-determination. Within these principles, residents should be centre stage, and this applies equally to the assessment process. Individuals need to be actively involved from the first day of admission and encouraged to have ownership of their care plan, which staff work consistently and collectively towards achieving. The outcome of assessment will be an improvement to the overall well being of the residents within the home.

Key points

- Avoid duplication of assessment by reading information already obtained.
- Assessment should support but not replace judgment.
- Assessment should help, and not be time-consuming.
- Assessment should measure what it purports to measure.
- Assessment and provision of help is continuous.
- Regular formal reviews are needed, rather than assessment being a 'one-off'.

CHAPTER 7

Doing things differently

Basic activities of daily living are carried out through a process of learning, which eventually develops into habits. For example, children are taught how to brush their teeth, comb their hair, get dressed and go to the toilet. After successfully managing tasks children internalise the processes and the tasks become almost automatic, and in many cases stand them in good stead for many years.

However, following the onset of physical and cognitive problems, when there is a dramatic reduction of functional abilities, this normal pattern of managing tasks can become seriously impeded. This can mean that people have to unlearn the way they have done things over potentially many years and then re-learn new ways of approaching things. Like any new skill, this can take a long time to master. It is important that this journey starts as soon as possible after the onset of loss of abilities, to avoid people learning inappropriate ways of coping. Inappropriate ways can cause the development of abnormal movement patterns.

It is possible to help residents become more independent by altering the way everyday activities are undertaken. A simple alteration of a technique can make an activity easier to do. This is based upon an approach that encourages and facilitates rather than direct care-giving or the provision of equipment and adaptations. By adopting different techniques, such as sliding rather than carrying items, breaking tasks into smaller parts, or sitting to do an activity rather than standing, residents can be helped to do as much as possible. By encouraging residents to use their physical and cognitive abilities to the full, their quality of life can improve. An enabling approach results in residents maximising their abilities and becoming more able to manage activities of daily living. However, new techniques can take time and much frustration before becoming easy.

When people are recovering from illness or becoming frailer, it is hard to watch them struggle with simple tasks. It is tempting to provide assistance or a piece of equipment to help minimise difficulties encountered in their everyday life. While in many circumstances this may be appropriate, it can be counterproductive – causing the unintended consequence of creating greater dependency. This may generate the need for additional help or more reliance on equipment and adaptations to undertake everyday activities. A reduction in independence for residents generates additional direct care responsibilities for staff. This is avoidable for some residents if a positive approach to care is adopted. To understand how to break this cycle of increasing dependency, it is important to appreciate how the body functions.

The amazing human machine

The human body is incredibly complex and is distinguished from mechanical machines by its amazing capacity to restore its own function and to overcome problems, even when a 'breakdown' occurs. By concentrating on building up stamina, strength and coordination, the body's restorative abilities improve. The 'best care' uses the inner strength of every individual to maximum effect. By focusing on improving the body's functions, individuals can learn to max- imise their abilities, leading to an improved capacity to undertake a wider range of tasks. This results in greater independence and enhanced self-confidence. A culture of care that focuses on the spiral of dependency can be translated into a care programme aimed at achievement, reward and satisfaction.

Ergonomics and anthropometrics

The starting point of adopting this type of programme is observing and assessing how individuals cope with their environment. This gives a greater understanding of individual needs. Ergonomics and anthropometrics are based on the average measurements of populations. Data provide us with an understanding of how individuals manage everyday activities. The International Ergonomics Association Executive Council (2000) defines ergonomics as:

> ... the scientific discipline concerned with the understanding of the interactions among human and other elements of a system, and the profession that applies theory, principles, data and methods to design in order to optimise human well-being and overall system performance.

Anthropometrics is defined as:

> ... the measurement of the dimensions of the body and other physical characteristics.

Anthropometrics applies to every aspect of daily life, for example: accommodation, product designs and even the positioning of a finished item. Data on the dimensions of a population remove guesswork from this aspect of design. However, everyone is different in shape and size, and as the body ages or develops physical restriction, an individual's ability to cope with the environment becomes affected. Although ergonomics and anthropometrics provide a benchmark, everyone is an individual – and the ideal height or method of doing a task for one person is not necessarily the same for another person.

Techniques of support

Failure to complete a task independently is often simply a result of only part of the task no longer being possible, not necessarily the whole of the task. Often, by simply altering the way a task is carried out, an activity can become easier to do and greater independence can be achieved. Examples of what to look out for, and techniques of support, include:

- Assess how far the individual can manage before assistance is needed.
- Analyse why that part of the activity is no longer possible.
- Check that all essential items are within reach.
- Try adopting a different technique, for example:
  - Encourage sitting when washing their face and hands instead of standing.
  - Encourage sliding items rather than lifting.
  - Encourage pushing up on the arms of the chair when rising.
- Supply only the minimum equipment necessary for the particular aspect of the task being undertaken.
- Look for any physical obstacles in the environment that are hindering the task.
- Analyse whether or not the tasks can be simplified or carried out in stages, particularly if fatigue is a problem.

Blockages

When observing people undertaking tasks, like personal care or domestic activities, it is possible to identify the blockages that prevent the completion of a task. These could result from physical problems or deficits of mental functioning. When the blockage is identified, concentrate on ways of overcoming this particular problem area. With experience, staff can analyse problem areas and come up with creative solutions. This may take the form of doing tasks differently, the provision of assistive equipment or making alterations to their environment.

Breaking activities down into component stages

Activities involving complex sequences of actions can be simplified by breaking the task into stages, perhaps concentrating on the last stage first. For example, when dressing, an individual may have difficulties managing cardigan fastenings. Instead of putting it on for him or her, staff should just help with the fastenings that the person has difficulty with.

Interlinked problems

Problem areas are often interlinked. For example: if someone has problems manipulating clothing when getting dressed, they are likely to have problems managing clothing and cleansing when toileting. Rather than concentrate on the activity, look at the interrelated physical problem. If a resident has problems with fine finger movements or has a weak grip, then work on this aspect in a recreational programme by designing activities with an emphasis on hand movements. Sometimes, a combination of different techniques and small assistive devices may be required. The two examples in Tables 7.1 and 7.2 illustrate this.

Finding the right solution

It is important to ensure that people function at the maximum level possible in every area of their lives, and to understand that everyone is an individual. By allowing people to attempt as much of an activity as possible, it helps use the body to the fullest extent. Providing effective help mainly involves facilitation and use of the skills and strengths that individuals have, rather than doing things for people. It is important to find the correct balance between helping people to do a task and allowing people to do activities for themselves. Providing too much help can impede the development of independence in functional

Table 7.1 Moving in bed and getting out of bed.

Find out which aspect of moving from lying to sitting with legs over the side of the bed is difficult.

- Try the other side of the bed, as it may be easier.
- Encourage the resident to use body momentum to assist with rising.
- Is the bed firm and high enough to rise easily from?
- Would a leg lifter, bed rails or mattress lifter help?

Table 7.2 Sitting to standing.

Encourage the resident to move forward slightly and place his or her arms on the armrests in preparation for standing. He or she should push up from the arms of the chair.

- Are chairs the right height for the resident? The correct seat height will range from 40.5–51 cm (16–20 in). Knees should be at 90°, allowing the thighs and buttocks to take equal weight.
- Is the seat base comfortable, yet firm?
- Are the armrests high enough to facilitate moving into a standing position from sitting?
- The resident's back should be well supported.
- There should be a gap of about 5 cm (2 in) from the back of the knee to the front edge of the cushion.

ability; conversely, providing insufficient help can mean individuals struggling unnecessarily. Getting this balance right is not easy, and care staff can be guided by treating therapists, but the overall approach should be agreed within a care plan.

Conclusion

There is no 'best' way of coping with a problem, so explore the options with your residents. What is a suitable solution for one person may be unacceptable for another; multiple choices should be provided. Often, the simplest solution is the most effective and the most difficult to find. Sometimes, just by exercising creativity and flexibility, problems can be overcome. There are, however times when physical alteration to the environment (Chapter 4) or assistive equipment, as detailed in Chapters 8–17 is required.

Key points

- Find out which part of the activity is the problem.
- Try to find an alternative way of achieving the activity.
- Work on the problem area in the activities programme.
- Provide assistive devices if these will achieve independence in a task.
- Continuously assess and review the activity.

CHAPTER 8

Assistive devices

Assistive devices are not new: for centuries, mankind has used tools and equipment to assist with everyday life. These were initially made from natural materials like wood, stone or even bone. Progress accelerated in the industrial age with the development of metal devices, the introduction of mass production and plastics, and more recently with the development of the microchip.

In society today, people are heavily dependent upon devices to help them manage their lives effectively. Gadgets and electrical labour-saving devices are used extensively within the home: can openers, blenders, vacuum cleaners and tools that assist with most aspects of life. Assistive devices, therefore, are commonplace.

The term 'assistive devices' includes any item, piece of equipment or product system used to increase, maintain or improve the functional capabilities of any individual experiencing problems with activities of daily living. Items can increase quality of life as well as improving the working environment. Assistive devices include equipment known as medical devices, community equipment and assistive technology. Items range from small items like padded handles on feeding utensils and bottle openers to hoists or profiling electric beds. They can be purchased, modified or customised.

Value of assistive devices

With technological advances, there are an increasing number of small assistive devices to enable residents to be self-sufficient or undertake activities that they wish to do more easily. Some items may only be required on a short-term basis, e.g. when recovering from illness, surgery or orthopaedic injuries. However, for some disabled people the provision of assistive equipment is essential to enable them to cope with the basic practicalities of life and overcome impairments of function. Older and disabled people and their carers have been the beneficiaries of an expansion of assistive equipment, and indeed there is a vast array of labour-saving devices available on the high street.

Sometimes there is a need for more specialist types of assistive equipment, specifically designed to help with particular tasks. However, some people refuse equipment as it will 'make them stand out', and if this is the case then individual preferences should be respected.

Disabilities are not just confined to the obvious physical ones, but include sensory impairment, such as partial hearing and sight, or cognitive and perceptual problems. Without the provision of an assistive device, an activity may be impossible and dependence on other people may be required. There can be a real sense of achievement in doing a task unaided, without the need for hands-on-care. Assistive devices are also available for leisure activities, ranging from playing-card holders to gardening aids to knitting and sewing devices. Several small assistive devices (Table 8.1) make an environment more accessible, make tasks easier and enable independence in some activities of daily living. Therefore it seems logical that the need for assistive devices will continue when people move into or from a care environment. However, many homes tend to focus just on mobility, bathrooms and feeding equipment.

Equipment in care homes

Responsibility for the provision of equipment by the public sector to care homes tended to be unclear for a number of years. However, Department of Health (2004b) guidelines state that '...people in local authority and private care homes have the same rights to services, including the provision of equipment, as those living in their own homes'. The principles behind provision include:

Table 8.1 Some general problems and solutions.

Problem	Solution
Problems signing documents or cards	Provide a clipboard Try different pens (larger, with non-slip grips) Ensure good task lighting (adjustable task lights, magnifying lights) Appropriate seating when writing
Difficulty bending down.	Use a lightweight long-handled reacher (pick-up stick)
Problems holding newspaper	Use a cantilever-type table with lip and tilting top and anti-slip surface or a book/newspaper holder
Unable to carry when using walking frame	Use clip-on net bag or shoulder bag Perhaps try a trolley or rolator (with integral bag) instead

- Loaned equipment should be properly maintained and returned promptly.
- Equipment must be issued as part of a risk management process, and staff must be competently trained.
- Guidelines state that if the NHS determines that an individual requires a particular piece of equipment, the NHS should do one of the following:
  - Ensure that the care home provides it
  - Provide it on a temporary basis until the care home is able to provide it, or
  - Provide it to the individual for as long as he or she needs it.

There are now 138 integrated community equipment services (ICES) in England able to 'loan' equipment out to individuals in a care home if the need for a particular piece of equipment 'falls outside of the home's general provision' (Table 8.2).

Table 8.2 Department of Health (2004b) guidelines on equipment provision.

Community equipment services should be willing, subject to local agreements, to help care homes wherever possible with the following (this will depend on local arrangements and resources):

- Advice on equipment.
- Staff training for equipment use and management.
- Equipment loans for individual users.
- Maintenance, testing and decontamination using specialist equipment.

Care managers should:

- Ensure that assessments meet Single Assessment Process and Fair Access to Care Services requirements and service user care plans make references to equipment needs as part of comprehensive/specialist assessments.
- Ensure that service users' needs are monitored and reviewed and that appropriate changes are made to care plans.

Care homes should be willing (subject to local agreements) to help community equipment services by:

- Checking ownership and arrangements for equipment when users are first admitted to the home
- Identifying when equipment is no longer required and releasing it promptly for collection
- Informing care managers of changes in service users' needs
- Informing the service promptly in the event of equipment breakdown
- Notifying changes in service user arrangements for whom equipment has been loaned (e.g. hospitalisation, movement to another care home).

The Department of Health (2004c) believes that it is unreasonable to expect care homes to provide individual items of equipment that are not used by other residents. This includes items that are specifically tailored (custom-made), perhaps by the design, size and weight requirements. However, guidelines state:

It is expected that care homes providing nursing care will be fit for purpose, which, in the main, means they will have in place basic handling, mobility and lifting equipment and adaptations.

ICES, therefore, do not generally provide items for 'common usage' (such as hoists, high-seated chairs and bath lifters).

To help understand this system, the Department of Health (2004c) has issued appendices containing 'flowcharts' to guide the reader through the eligibility criteria. It may be possible to obtain equipment to help with personal care from the integrated equipment service if it is to be for the resident's sole use. These guidelines are available electronically and can be printed off for reference.

Sources of advice

The Medical Devices Agency produces regular reports on comparisons of equipment and highlights adverse incidents. The Department of Health (2002c) states:

The Medicines and Healthcare products Regulatory Agency welcomes reports of adverse incidents about medical devices and equipment from anyone, regardless of whether they are an individual or work for an organisation.

The Disabled Living Foundation (DLF) helps people to locate items and provides impartial information on a wide range of equipment. The DLF's web site (DLF, 2006a) has several useful fact sheets on equipment, many of which were updated in 2006. They are helpful to identify sources of suitable assistive devices, e.g. Choosing Household Equipment (DLF, 2006b). The fact sheets provide many ideas on different techniques and assistive equipment. The DLF describe four types of equipment that are:

- designed specifically for older or disabled people to overcome a particular difficulty, e.g. a wheelchair, a bath board, or a raised toilet seat;
- standard equipment with a particularly helpful feature, e.g. an electric tin opener, vacuum cleaner, food processor or computer. All of these can take the physical effort out of an activity;

- standard equipment that has been adapted, e.g. an extension on a comb for a person with limited reach, or suckers on a nail brush for someone who has the use of only one hand;
- custom-made items specially designed for particular needs of one person.

It is important to give residents the opportunity to test out equipment, and some homes have a supply that residents can experiment with. It is useful to have a range of up-to-date equipment catalogues in stock for reference.

Larger and expensive items should be tried out first before purchase to assess their suitability. Manufacturers and agents will visit care homes to advise on products, and some equipment can be provided on a trial basis. Many exhibitions take place throughout the world to give opportunities to therapists, purchasers, carers and people with disabilities to get up to date with the bewildering range of equipment and to compare products. In the UK, Naidex and Independent Living run annual events open to professional staff and the general public.

There are over 50 disabled living centres in the UK that offer solutions to practical difficulties in daily living. They have a wide range of demonstration products and are normally staffed by occupational therapists providing the opportunity to try out different products. The centres provide unbiased expert advice and information about what is available, how much it costs and where to get it. Details of local centres are available electronically at `http://lut.ac.uk/info/usabilitynet/dlcc.html`.

Other sources of equipment

Although the sources of funding for equipment vary throughout the world, there is an increase in consumer independence and suppliers. There are many outlets for assistive devices, with some retailers selling a few specialist items while others stock hundreds of items. Several retailers sell 'kits', such as hip/knee equipment packages, at a discount. Sources of assistive devices include high-street chemists, local disability equipment stockists, mail order outlets, major distributors of assistive devices, and the Internet. Using the Internet, people can search and order products worldwide with a plethora of suppliers of equipment and multiple choice. Using Google and the search words '*equipment+disability*' produced 2,230,000 worldwide sites in April 2007. Although the Internet is a useful tool for researching, it can be time-consuming. The Yellow Pages are another good starting point.

Supermarkets sell household items that can be used by people with disabilities, such as hairbrushes with lightweight enlarged handles. Items designed to cope with a disability and which are provided for an individual's use are often VAT exempt. Declaration forms are available from equipment suppliers or retailers, and provide a discount of 17.5% off the cost of an item.

Custom-made pieces of equipment

Additional to 'off-the-shelf' products, specialised custom-made items may need to be made by manufacturers if a person's needs cannot be met by the existing range of equipment. The REMAP organisation (http://www.remap.org.uk/) provides individually made items for specific problem areas. REMAP has over 100 groups in the UK and welcomes new volunteers, particularly with skills in areas of design, manufacture and medical fields. Local schools or colleges will probably welcome the chance to have 'live' design projects. An example of this is a specialised telephone holder made by a school for attachment to a stand-up bed.

The London Metropolitan University has an MA course in Design Research for Disability (http://www.londonmet.ac.uk/courses/). Several of the students' innovative technologies and products are on the BBC web site (2005a). Examples of projects are:

- Postural seating to support disabled children after spinal or hip surgery
- Floor-to-ceiling bedroom drawer units on a revolving chain mechanism so that they can be reached from standing or a seated position
- User-friendly central heating timers with LEDs (light-emitting diodes) that have better colour-contrast, showing various on and off times on separate displays
- Telephones that dial automatically when a card is placed into a card/photo holder and the photo or holder is simply tapped.

Safe use of equipment

The Medical and Healthcare products Regulatory Agency (MHRA) have an interactive online education programme that is aimed at healthcare staff to increase their knowledge of regulations and the safe use of devices (http://www.mhra.gov.uk/home/idcplg?IdcService=SS_GET_PAGE&nodeId=51). In September 2005, independent and objective evaluation of medical devices previously under the MHRA was passed to the Centre for Evidence-based Purchasing (2005). All evaluation reports published since 2002 are now available electronically at `http://www.pasa.nhs.uk/PASAWeb/NHSprocurement/ CentreforevidencebasedPurchasing/CEPoutputs/LandingPage.htm`.

Residents moving out of care into the community

Some residents may be admitted for respite or reside in an intermediate care bed. If assistive devices may be required on discharge then contact the community occupational therapist or social services who will arrange for the provision of equipment. Items to help with bathing, toileting, dressing and feeding can be obtained.

In the UK, under the NHS and Community Care Act 1990 a local authority social services department has a duty to carry out assessments for people it believes to be in need of services and to assess disabled people. The Fair Access to Care Services (FACS) (Department of Health, 2003d) provides guidance on eligibility criteria based on the degree of risk an individual might face. These risks have been placed into four main categories: critical, substantial, moderate and low (Table 8.3).

Individual councils set their own level of eligibility for services based upon the FACS criteria. Many councils do not meet the needs of individuals who fall within the 'low' banding, although they will generally offer advice and guidance. In these circumstances, individuals will be responsible for accessing their own equipment and would be best advised to seek guidance if they are not certain what is available. However, many items are available on the high street to improve quality of life, and this is useful particularly as small items may not be provided from social services or the ICES store.

The trend in policy terms has been to develop a consumerist approach to care and equipment provision. Since the UK Prime Minister's Strategy Unit report *Improving the Life Chances of Disabled People* (NHS Purchasing and Supply Agency, 2005), the government proposes to increase the take-up of direct payments and to test other forms of individual budgets for people using local authority services. Direct payments (Department of Health, 2001b) enable individuals to buy in the services they need, e.g. respite care, carers and technology to assist in independent living (Table 8.4). Recommendations of the green paper include the development of new responsive models of care, including extra care housing and telecare, and a shift to more preventative services. The report says, 'independent living is about providing disabled people with choice, empowerment and freedom'. This will mean that the power of spending will shift more to individual purchasers of assistive equipment.

Table 8.3 Department of Health eligibility framework: four bands.

- **Critical**: When life is, or will be, threatened; and/or significant health problems have developed or will develop; and/or there is, or will be, little or no choice and control over vital aspects of the immediate environment; and/or serious abuse or neglect has occurred or will occur; and/or there is, or will be, an inability to carry out vital personal care or domestic routines; and/or vital involvement in work, education or learning cannot or will not be sustained; and/or vital social support systems and relationships cannot or will not be sustained; and/or vital family and other social roles and responsibilities cannot or will not be undertaken.

- **Substantial**: When there is, or will be, only partial choice and control over the immediate environment; and/or abuse or neglect has occurred or will occur; and/or there is, or will be, an inability to carry out the majority of personal care or domestic routines; and/or involvement in many aspects of work, education or learning cannot or will not be sustained; and/or the majority of social support systems and relationships cannot or will not be sustained; and/or the majority of family and other social roles and responsibilities cannot or will not be undertaken.

- **Moderate**: When there is, or will be, an inability to carry out several personal care or domestic routines; and/or involvement in several aspects of work, education or learning cannot or will not be sustained; and/or several social support systems and relationships cannot or will not be sustained; and/or several family and other social roles and responsibilities cannot or will not be undertaken.

- **Low**: When there is, or will be, an inability to carry out one or two personal care or domestic routines; and/or involvement in one or two aspects of work, education or learning cannot or will not be sustained; and/or one or two social support systems and relationships cannot or will not be sustained; and/or one or two family and other social roles and responsibilities cannot or will not be undertaken.

Misuse of assistive devices

The use of equipment should be considered, particularly when there are residual difficulties yet assistive devices are only one method of overcoming a problem. By discussion and observation, the physical or cognitive difficulties that prevent completion of a task can be identified. Often, by adoption of a different

Table 8.4 Recommendation 4.4: Supporting independent living (NHS Purchasing and Supply Agency, 2005).

Government departments 'should, by 2012, work towards a new approach to supporting independent living, which delivers support, equipment and/or adaptations in a way that:

- Addresses all aspects of needs for support and/or equipment or adaptations
- Is personalised according to individual need and circumstances
- Is underpinned by the principle of listening to disabled people and acknowledging their expertise in how to meet their needs
- Maximises the choice and control that people have over how their additional requirements are met
- Provides people with security and certainty about what level of support is available
- Wherever possible, minimises the disincentive to seek paid employment or to move from one locality to another
- Uses existing resources to maximise social inclusion.'

technique or making changes to the immediate environment (i.e. looking at the ergonomics and removal of obstacles), tasks can be achieved without an assistive device. Tasks can be carried out in many ways (Chapter 7) and individual preferences will need to be considered when solutions are found.

Inappropriate use of assistive devices can prevent full function from being returned after illness, injury or operation. Whilst it is initially necessary to protect and limit movement, it is vital to dispense with equipment as soon as safety allows, thus facilitating the maximum return of body function. An example of this is a person who has undergone a hip operation, perhaps to replace a worn hip joint from osteoarthritis. A high-seated chair, a toilet raise and a higher bed used in conjunction with long-handled dressing aids and a long-handled reacher will enable independence but not encourage full use of the body. The quadriceps (the large muscle above the knee) will not be fully used in the process of rising and sitting. This muscle may atrophy (shrink) and weaken, and a resident's walking capacity may be affected. If dependency on equipment occurs, full potential may not be realised. Therefore, although post-operatively it is important to restrict the range of movement, this should be followed by graded daily activities to prevent weakness. As the saying goes: 'Use it or lose it'.

All adjustable equipment must be altered to fit correctly or it can prove hazardous. Several assistive devices are adjustable in height and width. Items must be altered to fit the user if the item is for their sole use: e.g. a walking appliance or equipment for an *en suite*. A compromise will need to be reached if the item is to be used by multiple users in shared facilities (e.g. toilet frames, shower chairs and higher seated chairs). Bathboards/showerboards and inside bath seats should be adjusted to fit the baths. Bathlifters have suction pads on the base to prevent movement that should be secured before transfers are attempted.

Conclusion

Together with a programme of activity, assistive devices can ensure that individuals are functioning at their maximum level of abilities to enable a wide choice of activities and to maintain optimal quality of life. The following chapters concentrate on several aspects of daily living to make tasks easier with a combination of alternative techniques and assistive devices.

Key points

- Try alternative methods before supplying an assistive device.
- Obtain an up-to-date catalogue of assistive equipment for reference.
- A resident's choice is important where multiple solutions are available.
- Integrated Community Equipment Services may supply assistive devices for individual residents, but not for common use.

PART 4

Supporting individuals with their personal care needs

CHAPTER 9

Personal hygiene

Every day people undertake personal care tasks, including hair care, tending to nails, putting on makeup and shaving. Several activities are concerned with hygiene; others are connected with appearance. Often considerable time and energy is spent on these activities, particularly when preparing for an important event or going somewhere special. Many routines are satisfying in themselves and considered pleasurable 'pampering sessions' that provide a sense of general well-being and self-esteem. Indeed, a whole industry has evolved to keep up appearances, from the barber's shop offering shaves to the leisure spas providing total grooming experiences. In private, individuals develop their own personal routines to get themselves ready.

The ability to undertaking grooming develops in childhood and the activities involved are often taken for granted. However, the skills required to carry out several of the tasks involve complex physical and cognitive activities. Firstly, there has to be recognition that the task needs doing, and then individuals have to perform a complex sequence of events. Body manoeuvrability, muscle power, fine finger movements and good sensation are required for most personal care tasks. For example, combing hair requires fine finger coordination, the ability to know where your limbs are positioned and the ability to reach upwards. For other tasks, like applying make-up, then good vision and considerable dexterity are needed.

The starting point

As people age, or if there is an impairment of physical or cognitive function, difficulties can develop that result in problems accomplishing these tasks independently or safely. Most people learn compensatory techniques or adjust their routines, but for some people their capacity to do this is restricted and they may need some additional assistance. As part of a good care environment, attention to these activities is essential to ensure that residents have a quality of life that affords them dignity and self-respect.

■ Make no assumptions

It is important not to make assumptions about a resident's capabilities. Lack of interest in appearance could be due to treatable medical problems like depression. However, when a person neglects their appearance this may stem from struggling to manage tasks and not wishing to disclose problems, not necessarily as a result of indifference. Personal choice should be respected, unless specific medical or hygiene reasons shape the timing, frequency and methods used.

■ Individual needs

Staff will have some details of a resident's capabilities on admission to a home, but it is essential to get to know the individual resident and to establish individual needs, routines, preferences and capabilities. The assessment on admission should have revealed preferences, but obviously it is important to review and update assessments, as function can improve or deteriorate. Staff will observe and assess how residents cope with their personal grooming. The importance of accurate assessment is discussed in Chapter 6.

■ Routines

Adherence to past routines is important to help a person settle into a home. Find out from relatives and friends the previous lifestyle and routines, e.g. did they bathe, shower or have a strip wash? What time of the day did they bathe or shower? Establishing a regular routine can help, but as dementia changes all aspects of a person's life, it can also alter a person's approach to their appearance and habits of grooming.

Establish problem areas and ways of helping

Individuals may encounter problems with only part of the task; for example, a person may be able to brush the front part of the head but not the back. Sometimes this can be the first stage of the task, or it may be necessary for care staff to start the task and then hand over to the resident to complete. By allowing and facilitating the resident to do as much as possible, care staff help maintain self-esteem and skills. This gives residents a sense of being in control of their own body and life. A by-product is that a resident who actively participates in personal care tasks also benefits from the exercise that helps maintain physical function and provides some cognitive stimulation.

Problem areas are often interlinked, so rather than concentrating on the specific activity, look at the interrelated physical problem. For example, if a resident has problems with grooming tasks involving fine finger movements or weak grip, then design activities with an emphasis on hand movements as well as concentrating on the particular task that is problematic. Specific movements can be incorporated into the resident's activity programme utilising a mixture of group and individual activities.

By looking at how a resident copes with tasks, blockages can be identified and solutions sought. There are six main aspects to consider when providing assistance:

- Offering general advice
- Personal care assistance
- Using different techniques
- Assistive equipment
- Adaptations
- Environmental issues

Each of these is considered in turn.

I *Offering general advice*

Often guidance can resolve the problem, as people may struggle with an activity merely because they have not learned techniques to overcome specific problems. Using different techniques (Chapter 7) or more manageable clothes (Chapters 13 and 14) can help. The Disabled Living Foundation's (2006a) web site has a series of downloadable booklets on many aspects of personal care, including dressing, bathing and showering. Advice needs to take into consideration the individual's preferences and compromises may be needed. It is important to empower individuals to make the right choice for themselves. The key to providing a good service is to ensure that the advice provided follows an appropriate assessment that takes into account individual needs.

Any instructions should be clear and in a format that residents can understand, e.g. short phrases, words, gestures or even a demonstration of an activity. Although most grooming activities are carried out to cleanse and refresh they can be enjoyed as forms of relaxation if provided in a relaxed, unhurried atmosphere. A positive care staff approach to this task transforms mere tasks to a pleasurable pursuit. Care staff undertaking personal care activities can either allow residents to do as much of an activity as possible or they can increase dependency on staff. For some activities it is easier for busy staff to do the task for the resident, but this short cut should be resisted as much as possible.

2 Personal care assistance

It is important to remember that many personal care activities are normally private activities. Initially, there may be a sense of embarrassment, a feeling of disempowerment and loss of independence when care staff help with personal care activities. If embarrassment is the reason for refusing assistance then tact and persuasion are required. This often requires considerable sensitivity by staff, as the very nature of several activities means they are undertaken in private. Residents may find difficulty talking about personal care needs, so it is critical for staff to use their initiative.

Reluctance to accept assistance can be for many reasons. Overcoming this may be as simple as making sure the help is offered at the preferred time of day. People may want to continue with old habits; this should be respected and methods that are appropriate and safe for an individual should be encouraged. Assistance can be provided in a respectful and enabling way to minimise any potential distress. Approaching the subject in an understanding way is the best style. A good balance is needed between respecting privacy to being available to help.

3 Using different techniques

Different techniques can be used to facilitate activities (Chapter 7), perhaps using a different position, e.g. sitting to do a task may be easier than standing. Activities that involve complex sequences of actions can be broken down into their component stages and one aspect carried out by the resident. Proper planning of the task includes ensuring that all items required are at hand and laid out in accordance with the sequence of the task. This is particularly helpful for residents who may be confused or have cognitive or perceptual problems.

4 Assistive equipment

Although assistive equipment can help people manage personal care activities more easily, it is not advisable to provide assistive devices as the first option. Try altering the techniques or adjusting the environment, as these are more sustainable and satisfactory to individuals. However, some people require equipment, and residents with a longstanding or progressive disability may already have some items of assistive equipment when moving into a care environment. The Department of Health (2004b) states that Integrated Community Equipment Services (ICES) should be willing to help care homes wherever possible, but that this will depend on local arrangements, resources and budget constraints. Items provided by ICES should not be used communally. Items for communal use can be obtained from specialist companies or from local retailers such as chemists and supermarkets.

Assistive devices are broadly discussed in Chapter 8, with specific equipment dealt with under topic areas (e.g. bathing, showering and toileting in Chapters 10–12). The Disabled Living Foundation (2006a) provides an information service and fact sheets on many aspects of personal care. The items in Table 9.1 provide examples of the wide range of items currently available for washing, hair management, skin care and nail care. They are listed to give an indication of the range and are not endorsements of particular products or manufacturers. Several small assistive devices are available at high street shops, including chemists, ranging from long-handled combs to magnifying mirrors. Many everyday items for grooming are made from lightweight plastics; indeed several have chunky gripping surfaces that are useful for residents with poor grip.

Table 9.1 Items to help with personal care.

Activity	Items
Hair care	Long handled combs and brushes Enlarged grips for brush and comb handles Hair wash trays allow hair washing from a seated or lying position Hands-free hair dyer on a stand or held in a clip attached to a wall
Nail care	Nail brush or nail file on suckers Nail trimmers mounted onto a base with non-slip feet that clip nails with a push of the lever Scissors with enlarged hand grips, e.g. styrex scissors
Skin care	Use push down pump dispensers instead of screw top containers or items with tight lids Decant lotions into dispensers
Washing and 'strip washing'	Tap turners or lever taps to washbasins are easier when hand function is impaired Sensor operated soap dispensers Long-handled sponges and brushes Flannel back washers with loops at either end
Drying self	Towels with loops at either end Towelling dressing gowns Body/hand dryers.
Securing items if 'one-handed' user	Suction pads Non-slip surface, e.g. pimple rubber, non-slip mesh or Dycem

If short-stay residents need equipment to cope with daily living, it is essential that referral is made to the community services in good time to ensure that provision is available on discharge from care. Customers of rented properties may be able to take advantage of 'Fast track' minor adaptations undertaken by Housing Associations (for example handrails and lever taps) if this service is operational.

5 Adaptations

Adaptations to facilitate personal care tasks range from a single handrail to a complete refurbishment of the bathroom, *en suite* or toilet area. The Building Regulations (2000) provide guidelines on suitable room dimensions, circulation spaces and heights of fixtures, rails, lighting and pull cord alarm systems and are a useful reference point. Approved Document M – Access to and Use of Buildings published by the Office of the Deputy Prime Minister (2006) updates the Building Regulations (2000). When designing products and buildings, average limb lengths, height and range of movement (anthropometrics) are used. Chapter 4 discusses how care homes can be made more accessible.

6 Environmental issues

Environmental constraints can turn impairments of function into disabilities. Although building regulations can provide guidance on heights of fixtures, individual adjustments might need to be made, particularly if a resident has a physical impairment that affects range of movement. Generally speaking, if an inclusive design is followed this will cater for most disabilities, although minor repositioning of items like towel rails, toilet roll holders and mirrors may be required. To help with adjustment of clothing and grooming, mirrors should be viewable from a seated and standing position. A common mistake is to have several rows of tiling sited above the sink and then the mirror placed above, as this can exclude those who use wheelchairs. Mirror tiles could be used instead, or a tilting mirror installed.

Specific problem areas

In a residential care setting, personal care activities can pose particular problems for many residents, including:

- Finding the way
- Transferring into the bath or shower and on and off the toilet
- Temperature control
- Washing and drying the body
- Safety and alerting help

Several of these are related to the environment that the resident lives in and paying attention to detail can help make tasks easier for residents and carers to manage.

■ Finding the way

Signage is useful, but residents with visual problems may prefer contrasting pictorial images. Bathroom doors painted the same colour will help residents to differentiate bathrooms from other rooms. The 'pink' or 'blue' door is easier to find than the 'fifth door on the left'. General environmental issues are mentioned in Chapter 4.

■ Transferring into the bath or shower and on and off the toilet

Several assistive devices have dual uses for bathing, showering and toileting.

– *Handrails*

These provide additional support when moving from sitting to standing or transferring and can provide support when standing, e.g. to wash or to urinate. Smooth or ribbed (textured) handrails are available; a textured rail is easier to grip with wet hands. A contrasting rail is easier to see against a background. Plastic rails are quicker to install than metal, as they do not need earth bonding. ODPM (2006) provides details and diagrams of recommended handrail positions. Guidelines are useful, but individual anthropometrics should be applied; for example, looking at the reach and hand function of individuals.

– *Floor-to-ceiling poles*

Vertical poles can help with standing and balancing when a carer is helping with clothing. However, poles can impede transfers, particular when using a bathlifter or bathboard, as they can restrict access beside a bath.

■ Temperature control

Bathing has been associated with a high number of reported fatal or serious scalding incidents and safe water temperatures are essential. Temperature control is therefore very important when considering hand washing, bathing and showering. The National Minimum Standards (Department of Health, 2003b) emphasises that water temperatures should be at maximum limits to ensure safe practices in nursing and residential care homes. Standard 25.8 states: 'To prevent risks from scalding, pre-set valves of a type unaffected by changes in water pressure and which have fail-safe devices are fitted locally to provide water close to 43 °C'. Many showers have 'temperature locks' that ensure that the temperature of the water is 40 °C. Several manufacturers produce 'smart' plastics that change colour if the temperature is over 37 °C or 47 °C. Floating thermometers can be used rather than a subjective 'elbow test'. Shower units must be thermostatically controlled to avoid a change in water temperature.

■ Washing and drying the body

Single-action lever taps are easier to manage and taps can be operated by sensor controls. However, both cross and crystal taps can be operated using a tap turner that effectively converts taps to lever operation. Rather than change the whole tap, lever conversion kits can be purchased, but these are similar in price to a new lever tap. Check that the towel holder is sited within reach of ambulant and wheelchair users from the washbasin and toilet. The provision of a perching or shower stool by the washbasin is of benefit for resident who have a limitation of standing ability or poor balance. In communal areas, paper towels or hot air dryers are more hygienic than towels. Hand or body dryers can be strategically placed to enable independent drying.

■ Safety and alerting help

The hard, smooth surfaces in a bathroom, shower room, toilet or *en suite* can become dangerously slippery when wet and falls can occur. A hazard warning should be put in place if the floor is wet, to alert other users. The provision of slip-resistant flooring and bath mats is recommended. Additional slip-resistant shapes can be used in the bath or on the rim of the baths to give greater stability. Both need replacing on a regular basis. Staff should never leave a confused mobile patient unattended during bathing. Red alarm cords must be placed within a resident's reach while in the bath, with red bangles placed at 100 mm and 800 mm to 1000 mm above floor level (ODPM, 2006).

Some problem areas

There is no ideal or best way of overcoming any particular problem. Solutions need to be tailored to individual needs, so it is important to explore the options with individual residents. The following outlines some problem areas and offers practical solutions to illustrate what can be done.

■ Wheelchair user

Before admission, check that there is sufficient space for turning and transfer within the resident's room and *en suite*. Ensure that there is space to get close to tables, drawer units and the sink. A wheelchair user will have problems gaining access to high or low cupboards and units. Place items like soap, flannel and denture containers within reach. Sliding doors are easier to access.

■ Difficulty standing for any length of time
Problems with standing can arise from loss of energy, general tiredness, pain, shortness of breath, weakness, back conditions, unsteadiness and balance impairments. Residents may be unable to stand to groom themselves and a chair or stool can assist in conjunction with accessible mirrors.

■ Difficulty bending down to lower legs and feet
Many residents cannot reach down to their feet due to back, hip problems or obesity. Being unable to reach the feet causes problems with dressing, foot care, and washing and drying legs and feet. Long-handled assistive equipment can help.

■ Limitation of reach
Limitation of upper arm movements or weakness due to neck or shoulder problems causes difficulties reaching and with activities such as feeding, washing, teeth and hair care. Long-handled equipment can assist.

■ Impaired function in one arm
Many medical conditions, for example, a stroke or a severe head injury, can cause a reduction of function down one side of the body. This can result in as much impairment as an amputated arm or hand. Items will require stabilising and need to be operated by one hand only, and different techniques will be needed.

■ Incoordination and tremor
Multiple sclerosis and cerebellar tumours are two medical conditions that affect coordination. Parkinsonism often produces a fine rest tremor. Many factors can increase problems, such as stress, anxiety, fatigue even the consumption of caffeine. Weighted handles may help control a fine tremor. Stabilising the arm on a table/worktop can give additional control and support. It is essential to assess the resident with any items that might cause injury due to tremor, e.g. combs.

■ Weakness of grip or painful hands
Rheumatoid arthritis causes painful swollen joints that result in weakness of grip. Weak grip can be due to general frailty, disuse or one of many clinical conditions that affects muscle power including motor neurone disease. Lightweight enlarged easy-to-use grip handles on grooming aids can be purchased.

■ **Impairment of fine finger movements**

This can stem from conditions affecting the central nervous system or individual nerves in the arm and hand. It causes problems with any activity requiring dexterity. Picking up small objects, e.g. a tail comb, may be difficult and an enlarged handle can be attached.

■ **Loss of visual field or impaired vision**

Problems with vision can occur due to damage or deterioration of the eyes, impairment of perception or cognitive problems. In addition to blurred vision, residents may have a loss of their visual field and, for example, may be unable to see to one side (hemianopia) or have loss of central vision. Attention, therefore, should be paid to the environment. Try to put all items back in the same place or in the same order. If there is signage on the resident's door ensure that they can identify this; a picture or a sheet of plain coloured paper may be easier to locate than a number or name plate.

■ **Communication problems**

Problems with hearing or understanding speech can be profound. It is vital to ensure that residents understand what is being said. Alternative communication methods may be required, such as using gestures or giving physical prompts; for example, passing a toothbrush to them.

■ **Perceptual and cognitive problems**

Strokes, head injuries and brain tumours can cause perceptual deficits and impairment of cognition, as can dementia. Residents may not recognise an everyday object (agnosia) or encounter problems knowing what to do with an object (apraxia). They may not be able to cope with new learning, but retain old routines (e.g. they may be able to manage the older type of screw top toothpaste but not the newer stand up dispenser). Residents with cognitive impairment may have forgotten the sequence of carrying out a task and require prompting. Try to keep items near where the activity should be carried out: e.g. comb, brush or makeup near the mirror, toothpaste and toothbrush together. Wherever possible, break activities down into stages and provide clear instructions.

■ **Behavioural issues**

Often, by looking at the antecedents to behaviour, the behaviour itself and the consequence of the actions, it is possible to find reasons for behavioural problems. This is easy to remember as the ABC of behaviour (A = antecedent, B = behaviour, C = consequence). Observing and talking to residents can identify problem areas. Verbal and non-verbal communication may be needed to ensure that residents understand. Some of the problems shown in Table 9.2 may apply to residents. Using distraction techniques, such as chatting or activity, is useful, as is shown in this example by Bonner (2005):

At changeover, the carers are complaining about how aggressive Mrs J is when being showered. A junior carer pipes up, 'I don't have any trouble. I ask her to turn on the water, which I adjust, and I give her the soap while I use another cake'.

■ Time of day and medication

The activity may be easier to manage at another time of the day, or the timing of medication could be altered to make carrying out the activity easier; for example medication to cope with the 'on–off' phenomenon if present (refer to Chapters 28 and 29 on Parkinsonism), or painkillers for rheumatoid arthritis.

Table 9.2 Problems with personal care activities and possible solutions.

■ Can they remember the processes?
Provide verbal and visual prompts – e.g. gather up all the items and guide the resident during the activity.
■ Do they recognise and know how to use the products and facilities?
Do not bombard with items, but give one item at a time in the right sequence, therefore providing prompts
(They may have agnosia or apraxia)
Keep dangerous substances e.g. cleaning solutions out of reach.
■ Perhaps they don't want to have another person look at them.
Tact, sensitivity and persuasion are required.
■ Do they have sufficient mobility and balance?
Provide suitable equipment.
Place toiletries within reach.
Ensure all fixtures in *en suites* are within reach.
■ Are they reluctant to bathe?
Maybe they prefer to have a strip wash. Provided they are happy with this method, this should be respected.

Conclusion

A combination of trying different methods and the provision of assistive equipment may enable residents to manage part or all of an activity. Often greater independence can be achieved by altering the way a task is carried out, but the simplest and most effective solution is the most difficult to find. Keeping up appearances is important, as it has an impact on an individual's sense of well-being, irrespective of age. A positive approach to this aspect of personal care is vital to ensure that residents enjoy as fulfilled a life as is possible and independence should be encouraged and prolonged for as long as possible. Success in tasks enhances independence and provides personal dignity.

Key points

- Many residents experience difficulties with activities of daily living.
- Environments can help or hinder the activity.
- Alteration of a technique can make an activity easier to do.
- A combination of alternative techniques and assistive equipment may be needed.
- Personal care activities can be used as forms of relaxation or enjoyment.
- Make personal care activities pleasurable by adopting a facilitative and positive approach.

CHAPTER 10

Washing bodies

Washing is part of a personal care routine that has many facets. Although the main reasons for washing are to avoid body odour and to maintain good skin condition, cleansing can be a positive experience, used as a form of relaxation or enjoyment which provides time to relax.

Individuals develop their own personal preferences for washing their bodies: some enjoy long soaks or quick dips in a bath, while others prefer a shower or a strip wash. Several residents entering care homes may not have experienced showering and may prefer to either bathe or have a strip wash, and this should be respected. Attempts at trying to persuade someone to shower, bathe or wash in the morning may be met with resistance if previously this was an evening activity.

Problems with washing

Many residents need help to access a bath or shower and have problems reaching parts of their bodies. However, with the provision of some long-handled equipment they may be enabled to wash all or part of their body. To reduce risks of cross infection, items should not be communal or stored in shared bathrooms. Items useful in *en suites*, if bathing or showering facilities are provided, include long-handled or larger-grip equipment. Examples are:

- A long-handled brush and sponge or back washer, if reaching is difficult.
- A wash mitt, if gripping is a problem.
- Suction nailbrushes, if grip is weak or the resident can only use one hand.
- Drying can be difficult due to loss of dexterity or restricted range of upper limb movement, but a long piece of webbing can be attached to one end of a towel or a wash strap can be obtained.

Washing hands

It is part of good hygiene to encourage residents to wash their hands before and after eating. It is very difficult to give your hands a good wash if you only have the use of one hand or have a limited reach, loss of handgrip or poverty of movement. Try the examples in Table 10.1 to find out how difficult tasks can be.

■ **Gaining access to the sink**
The use of a wheelchair or a walking aid can impede access to the sink, particularly if waste bins are in the way, so ensure hazard-free passage is possible.

■ **Turning the taps off and on**
To operate a crystal or capstan type tap requires coordination and sufficient range of movement in joints and grip. Several retailers stock detachable tap turners that help with tap turning; alternatively, the top of the tap can be replaced with a lever action tap (conversion kit). However, the cost of a conversion kit is around the same price as a new set of lever action taps. Push-down taps can be difficult for elderly frail people to manage. Sensor taps only deliver water when the sensor beam is crossed, thus reducing water consumption and also the chance of sinks overflowing. Many sinks in public places have sensor taps and these would be of use in care homes.

Table 10.1 An activity to try: washing hands.

1. Go to the washbasin and wash your hands.
2. Now try to wash your left hand without any assistance from your right hand.
3. Repeat this from a wheelchair position.
4. Repeat this simulating a loss of grip and then a loss of dexterity.

Could you:

■ Gain access to the sink?
■ Turn the taps off and on?
■ Reach the soap?
■ Wash your hands?
■ Reach towel/paper towel/hot air dryer and dry your hands?

What problems did you encounter?
What problems will your residents experience?
How can these problems be minimised?

- **Reaching the soap**

The soap dispenser should be within reach and able to be managed by the resident. Some soap dispensers need a two-handed operation: one hand to stabilise the dispenser whilst the other hand pushes down the plunger. This, of course, is very difficult for a person who only has the use of one hand.

- **Washing hands**

A suction nailbrush that is attached to the sink by suction cups is available to help one-handed people.

- **Reaching towels etc**.

Often drying devices are out of reach of wheelchair users, so ensure that they are all within reach.

- **Managing dentures and cleaning teeth**

Suction nailbrushes can also be used to clean dentures. Extracting toothpaste can be frustrating, but there are several toothpaste tube squeezers for one-handed use. Consider using a battery-operated toothbrush.

Cognitive and perceptual problems

It is likely that some residents will have cognitive or perceptual problems, in addition to physical problems, that may cause difficulties with washing and grooming. Residents who have cognitive problems will have problems with the sequence of washing and grooming, and may not do a task in the right order. They often display minimal organisational skills and will need reminding about their personal hygiene. They may also require prompting when carrying out tasks like washing hands and cleaning their teeth.

Residents who have perceptual problems may not be able to recognise, identify or name an object (agnosia), or may know what an object is and be able to describe how to use it but will not be able to perform the task (apraxia). The principles of task simplification can be utilised and tasks broken down into clearly defined stages so that one aspect is concentrated on. This may be at any stage in the process; for example the sink is filled, a flannel 'soaped', and the flannel then handed to the resident, or the resident could be asked to rinse the flannel out. Although staff may be able to multi-task, a resident who is 'cognitively or perceptually challenged' may only be able to concentrate on one aspect of a task.

Many of the principles of making the environment easier for residents to cope with that are applied elsewhere in this book can be applied with any task, particularly with personal care. For example, ensure that the items used contrast with the background. Residents who have perceptual, visual or cognitive problems will have problems identifying white soap in a white sink or a cream towel held in a cream towel holder against a cream wall. Many retailers sell bathroom accessories that are in bright primary colours and soap is available in all colours. By applying a principle of using strong contrasting colours (coloured soap and towels that contrast against walls) and generally de-cluttering the immediate environment tasks will be easier for the resident to carry out.

Whatever method of cleansing is chosen staff and residents should not be at risk and safe practices should be followed:

Risk assessment

The Manual Handling Operations Regulations (Department of Health, 1992), which came into force on 1 January 1993, state that risk assessment is vital and policies and procedures on moving and handling must be followed. HSE (2006) define that a risk assessment is:

> ... simply a careful examination of what, in your work, could cause harm to people, so that you can weigh up whether you have taken enough precautions or should do more to prevent harm

and

> The law does not expect you to eliminate all risk, but you are required to protect people as far as 'reasonably practicable'.

A risk assessment must be 'suitable and sufficient' and 'you need to be able to show that:

- A proper check was made;
- You asked who might be affected;
- You dealt with all the obvious significant hazards, taking into account the number of people who could be involved;
- The precautions are reasonable, and the remaining risk is low; and
- You involved your staff or their representatives in the process.'

HSE provides a risk assessment template (http://www.hse.gov.uk/risk/template.pdf). If a person is to be left to manage unassisted, or is at risk of falling, then a risk assessment of his or her abilities should be undertaken, documented and regularly reviewed. A confused mobile person should never be unattended during bathing or showering and risk assessment should include a resident's management of the immediate environment.

Ensuring safety – correct manual handling

Human beings are not static loads and watery environments can turn them into slippery objects, requiring extra care to handle and control. More than a third of all injuries lasting over three days reported each year to the Health and Safety Executive (HSE) are caused by manual handling (HSE, 2004). The HSE (2004) booklet *Getting to Grips with Manual Handling* is based upon the 1992 Manual Handling Operations Regulations, which were amended in 2002. This short guide applies to a wide range of manual handling activities, including lifting, lowering, pushing, pulling and carrying.

The HSE (2006) outline how to assess the risks in your workplace by following five steps:

Step 1: Identify the hazards
Step 2: Decide who might be harmed and how
Step 3: Evaluate the risks and decide on precaution
Step 4: Record your findings and implement them
Step 5: Review your assessment and update if necessary

Manual handling should therefore be kept to a minimum and it is important that manual handling assessments include assessment of bathing and showering needs. Although it can be quicker to manually handle residents, repeated lifting can cause orthopaedic problems that may not materialise until many years later.

Individual moving and handling risk assessments should always be undertaken and recorded when physical assistance is needed. Specific guidelines should be referred to and a copy kept accessible by staff, for example located in the rooms in which it is to be used, such as the bathroom and residents' rooms, not just in the office.

There are a number of issues to consider, ranging from choosing the right equipment, controlling the environment and providing suitable training for staff. Staff need to be guided through good practice and be taught to use equipment safely. It is important for care staff to know how to move people safely using correct manual handling techniques. All care staff should be trained in manual handling and a 'no-lifting' preferred policy adopted, although this is not a legal requirement in the UK. Correct techniques should be followed by care staff when using assistive equipment with residents to ensure that safe transfers are possible, and this should be reflected in the care home's policies and procedures.

Cultural considerations

It is really important for staff to be aware of individual cultural heritage, particularly in relationship to what are often considered to be intimate activities, such as washing, dressing and cleansing after toileting.

Conclusion

Many personal care activities are not without hazard. In assisting residents to wash, it is important that attention is given to at least three issues: individual preferences, controlling and adapting the environment and ensuring that staff adopt a positive approach to a very personal activity. By doing this, it is possible to make personal care activities safe and pleasurable, particularly with the wide range of equipment currently available. Within the home, attention needs to be paid to the practical environment by designing the living space to best effect. It is particularly important to ensure that residents' cultural needs are met and care staff must preserve individuals' dignity.

Key points

- Assessment that takes into consideration a person's future needs is vital.
- Try things out as this will highlight problem areas and generate ideas to resolve them.
- Assistive equipment can prolong independence in washing.
- Risk assessments are essential in determining safety in washing practices.
- Establish individual needs and make no assumptions.
- Use building regulations as a template for public and communal areas.
- Use visually contrasting materials to aid identification of fixtures.

CHAPTER 11

Bathing

Some elderly people recall that bathing used to consist of a tin tub located in the kitchen, filled with water that was heated on the coal fire or on a 'black leaded' stove: showers did not exist. In modern homes, there is normally a choice of a bath or shower installed, with older properties converted to accommodate this. Most care homes have baths and showering facilities; therefore, personal preferences can be met and individual routines maintained.

For many residents, there is nothing that can replace a long soak in a bath. Bathing is a pleasurable experience and there is nothing like a long soak in a bath to unwind, to enjoy the buoyancy of water, to contemplate or to simply to let the mind wander. Bathing is therefore, not just about cleansing, it can be a time for relaxation and indulgence. Time should be given to residents to allow them to enjoy the experience. However, showers provide a more hygienic method of cleansing, particularly if a resident suffers from incontinence: a quick shower could precede a longer bath.

Bathing can be also be medicinal, particularly if preparations are used, although care is needed as perfumed bath preparations can irritate the skin. Simply applying cream after a bath can be therapeutic, perhaps to sooth aching limbs. However, Nazarof (2005a) notes that 'prolonged soaks in a bath can lead to macerated skin' and advises on products to use to prevent skin damage.

Preferably, baths should be sited to allow access at either side by a wheelchair or a carer, with room to allow hoisting, if needed. Manufacturers produce several different types of baths, including baths with integral lifting devices and specialised baths for disabled people. Table 11.1 gives an outline of some of the many baths available. Removing a bath or shower and installing another can be expensive and with an increasingly frail care home population, it is advisable to ensure that the facilities cater for dependent residents. A care home can invest in 'assistive baths' only to discover that a standard bath with strategically placed handrails and a removable bath lifter would have suited the residents more effectively, and would have been cheaper.

Table 11.1 A guide to some of the different baths available.

- **Standard bath**

Adaptable for people with many disabilities, using equipment like bath-boards, bath seats, bathlifts, floor fixed bath hoists, lever taps and hand-rails. No major adaptations are required. Fibreglass baths will split if a bath seat is used unless a 'hanging' seat is obtained.

- **Low (shallow) baths**

Less leg movement is needed to step in but the bath rim is too low to be of any support and lowering to the water level is difficult, but a bath seat can be used.

- **Step-in baths and walk-in baths**

Less lower limb mobility is required to access and most have an integral seat. The step can cause access problems for people with lower limb problems or wheelchair users. However, some seat units slide forward to avoid the need to manage the step.

- **Baths with integral bathlifts**

Several have seats that allow easy sideways transfer for a wheelchair user. Additional seating strapping is available. Reduces the need for moving and handling.

- **Rising baths and high–low baths**

Residents are transferred onto a platform and the filled bath then rises. They are larger than an average bath and should be installed with good clearance at either side to facilitate transfers and to prevent trapping of limbs when the bath is moving. They can be used with a hoist to reduce the need for moving and handling. Carers do not need to bend down to assist with washing; therefore back strain is avoided. The top can also be used as a changing plinth.

- **Tilting baths**

These permit sideways transfer at one side; then the door is closed and the bath fills and tilts. A hoist can be used, reducing manual handling and enabling residents to bath easily and safely.

Equipment used to assist with bathing

Safety is important and residents may need to be supervised at all times when bathing. Correct moving and handling procedures should be followed and assistive devices can make transfers safer for residents and staff. All equipment should be regularly checked and the manufacturer's service schedules should be maintained.

There are many different forms and combinations of assistive equipment that can be used to facilitate transfers in and out of the bath. The DLF (2006c) has a fact sheet on choosing a bath and bath accessories. The following are the most common items:

■ **Rails attached to the taps**

Although these provide security when stepping into a bath, they should not be used to pull up on or to rise from the bottom of the bath. Taps are not designed to take body weight. Detachable rails can impede transfers in and out of the bath and integral bath rails or wall-fixed rails are safer.

■ **Floor-fixed rails**

Although these are safe and secure they can impede transfers. Rails should be slip-resistant.

■ **Wall-fixed grab rails**

Rails are useful to provide a secure support when standing up, when sitting down in the bath or when a bath lifter is in operation. The wall must be able to support the weight of the user. Metal rails should be earthed by an electrician or suitably coated by the manufacturer.

■ **Bathboards**

Bathboards fit on the top of the bath across its widest width and can be used with a bath seat. Some boards are slatted or have drainage holes to allow use as a shower board and to be dried upon. Following several adverse incidents, apertures must now be less than 8 mm or more than 75 mm (Medicines and Healthcare products Regulatory Agencies, 2003) to avoid skin becoming trapped. Several have handgrips to assist with balance and transfers.

■ **Bath seats**

These enable a person to sit about halfway down a bath, at the water level. They can be freestanding or wedged into the sides of the bath. Care is needed, as some baths (of fibreglass construction) may split unless a 'hanging', suspended bath seat is installed. Although they provide a sitting surface, full immersion is impossible unless the seat is removed and replaced to assist egress. They are often used in conjunction with a bathboard.

■ **Bathlifts**

Standard baths can accommodate removable powered bathlifts that raise and lower the user out of the water. Most are battery powered and several have side flaps to assist safe transfer and avoid flesh being trapped. It is possible to have custom-made larger flaps to accommodate wider baths. They transport a person from the top of the bath to below the water level and it is important that the bathlifter takes the user from the bottom to the top of the bath. A safety strap provides added security when the bathlift is moving. A vertical rail will give stability when a carer is helping with washing and security when the bathlift is operating. Various controls are available to suit impaired handgrip.

■ **Shallowbaths**
These are lightweight resin 'baths' with drainage plugs, which fit over a standard bath. They are suitable for children or adults and raise the person higher than when using a normal bath and equipment.

■ **Bath steps and step stools**
These are rarely recommended, as the problem of getting down to the water level still arises and a bathboard and bath seat will provide a safer method of accessing.

■ **Hoists**
Many baths are designed to allow either 'end-on' or side access by a portable hoist, or it may be possible to remove a bath panel. However, a dripping hoist sling can be a safety hazard on flooring. There are several types of hoisting device to deal with varying degrees of immobility that provide considerable choice, i.e. mobile, floor fixed or ceiling track hoists. Ceiling tracks are useful if space is limited, as they can transfer a user from the bed to the bath to a chair, and the ceiling track can extend into a shower area. They can be used in conjunction with a dressing/shower platform. Slings must be compatible with the hoist used.

■ **Leg lifters**
These are made from strong webbing loops that are hooked over a foot and used to lift the leg over the bath (and bed) whilst the user is sat on a bathboard. They are useful for residents who want to bathe independently but have difficulty getting their legs over the side of the bath.

■ **Equipment to assist with washing**
There are many assistive devices on the market, including ones available in shops and supermarkets as well as specialist equipment outlets. Items include long-handled washing aids and suction brushes and are discussed in Chapter 10.

■ **Equipment to assist with drying**
Towels can have loops added to the ends if grip is poor. There are several hand, feet and body dryers available that can be used in communal or *en suite* bathrooms to help residents dry themselves without help. Some retailers sell

dressing gowns that are designed for wheelchair users with less fabric at the back of the garment.

Conclusion

There are many different baths and types of assistive equipment available. These help people to access a bath and enable carers to assist in a safe manner. The type of bath chosen depends on many factors, including the residents' level of mobility, the layout of the bathroom and available finance. Whatever the needs, there is always a suitable solution to meet them.

Key points

- There are many different types of bath.
- The range of assistive equipment is extensive.
- Long soaks and some bath products can harm the skin.
- Ensure that correct moving and handling procedures are followed.
- Not all assistive baths are suitable for people with physical disabilities, so care is needed with purchase.

CHAPTER 12

Showering

Showering as a preferred method of cleansing in the UK is a fairly recent phenomenon, and even people aged in their 50s and 60s would have been brought up in households where having a bath was the usual way of cleaning. Today, showers are more commonplace, whether sited over the bath or in a separate cubicle. Technology has expanded substantially, with easily controlled temperature settings for the water and lever handles for simple operation. Many modern power showers have multi-directional water sprays of different forces and are sited in environments with wall-to-wall, ceiling-to-floor tiling, producing a 'wet-room'.

Using a modern shower is more hygienic and more economical than taking a bath, as the water is fresh and less water is used. Showering is also safer and quicker than bathing. But despite the obvious advantages to having a shower, within a care home there are particular issues to be considered, as with any personal care activity. Shower units must be thermostatically controlled to avoid a change in water temperature, for example when water pressure falls if water is diverted to another part of the home. Many showers have 'temperature locks', to avoid scalds, that ensure the temperature of the water is under 40 °C.

Types of shower

There are many different types of shower, but what is suitable for one home is not necessarily suitable for another home or group of residents. Level-access showers and cabinets (Table 12.1), however, cater for all mobility requirements as they avoid the need to negotiate a step. In *en suite* showers, handrails and a folding shower seat are recommended, with all washing items within reach of the individual user.

■ Shower over the present bath

A shower can be installed over a bath and used in conjunction with a bathboard, bathlifter or floor-fixed hoist. This will, of course, depend on the resident's abilities to transfer and maintain a sitting balance. Bathlifters (Chapter 11) transfer a user into and out of the bath and provide a seat to shower and dry from. A bath or

Table 12.1 Level access shower facilities.

Examples of level access showers

- Neatdek 3 from Neaco (`http://www.neaco.co.uk/`)
- Aquabeau range from Boundary Bathrooms (`http://www.boundary-bathrooms.co.uk/`)

Examples of level access shower cabinets

- Sandwell MK 3 from Chiltern Invadex Ltd (`http://www.chilternin-vadex.co.uk/`)
- Synergy from Armitage Shanks (`http://www.armitage-shanks.co.uk/`)

---

shower board placed at the shower end of a bath enables users to sit and shower and be dried without transferring out of the bath. Fixed shower screens on a bath rim can impede transfers and a shower curtain is preferable.

- **Wet rooms or shower areas**

Wet rooms or large shower areas have the advantage of space. Most can accommodate a fixed shower seat, a shower chair and a shower stool, but a larger area is needed for a shower trolley. A half-wall by the shower area will act as protection from water for carers or portable screens can be used and will help to channel water. A shower floor can be laid to a fall (a gradient running away from the dry area to enable water drainage into a waste pipe or channel) making it into a 'wet room' using slip-resist tiling, resin or a specialised floor

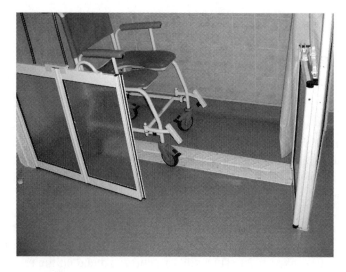

Wet room with equipment (© Julie Swann 2007).

covering. It is important to provide sufficient room for the carer to assist with washing without adopting an awkward or unsafe posture.

■ Shower cabinets

Shower manufacturers have, over time, recognised access problems that wheel-chair users or people with limited mobility encounter. Rather than having to sink a shower tray and put 'duckboards' over, level-access (wheeled-access) bases have evolved that avoid the need to negotiate a step and wheeled shower chairs can be used. Several cabinets can be fitted in place of a bath. Many shower cabinets have level access with a 'stable' door at the front or side to enable carers to assist without getting wet in the process. Some cabinets have integral seats or swing-out seats to facilitate transferring onto a wheelchair after the person is dried. The DLF (2003) fact sheet outlines choosing a shower and shower accessories.

■ Shower tray

High shower bases can be replaced with a lower-height tray or level-access tray. If drainage is a problem, waste pumps can be fitted externally (some are integral to a unit). Often, shower cabinets have a high step and a shower step with a slip-resistant surface will help a resident to the shower and an additional handrail may be required for safety. The handrail can be a floor to ceiling pole or wall hung depending on the structure of the shower walls.

Additional equipment for showering

■ Handrails

Strategically placed wall-fixed hand rails within reach can help the user into a standing position and give stability. Handrails will help residents to step into a shower cabinet and to maintain balance. Some cabinets have solid plastic sides and wall fixing is not possible, but a floor-to-ceiling pole may assist.

■ Shower seats

These can be fixed to a solid wall and many can be folded away when not in use. Some have integral armrests and can be adjustable in height for individual residents. Shower seats can be fixed to a solid wall, but a 'spreading plate' (load-bearing plate) may be required. If shower seats cannot be wall-fixed, a freestanding shower stool or chair may be required.

■ **Shower controls**

These should be easily reachable from a seated position and from the carer's position.

■ **Shower chairs**

These can be static or wheeled into the shower area, reducing the need for transferring into the shower area. Porcelain and modern acrylic bases will support most shower chairs; however, if bariatric equipment is used, it is advisable to check that the shower base will take the weight of a chair and resident.

■ **Half height shower doors**

Carers will need some form of water protection if assistance is given. Port-able and fixed half height shower screen can be provided if there is a wet room. Shower cubicles can be obtained with a half height door and side panel.

■ **Shower trolleys and showering plinths**

These are very useful for frail or severely disabled people. Assistance is given at the carer's waist height and bending is avoided. All have drainage holes and can be used in conjunction with hoists. They can double as a 'dressing table' and sluice facilities can be provided.

■ **Storage for items**

There are many wall-fixed storage units that can be obtained on the high street to contain shampoo, conditioner, shower gel and back washers or any other items that will be used. It is essential to have all items that a resident will use within reach so that they can access them independently.

■ **Hoists**

Wet, slippery bodies are difficult to handle and control. Staff should avoid lifting and handling, particularly as there are many assistive devices on the market specifically designed for enabling bathing and showering, for example portable and ceiling track hoists.

Individual preferences

Residents may dislike water on their face, in which case their hair can be shampooed separately from the showering (or indeed bathing) activity. Individual preferences need to be catered for and whatever individuals experienced before admission, opportunities should be given for various methods of cleansing.

Conclusion

It is important to appreciate that whilst showering is not a hazard-free activity, steps can be taken to minimise the risk to residents and to staff. Obviously, allowing residents the opportunity to have a shower may lead to them preferring this method of cleansing, but the point is that individual choice is allowed.

Key points

- Showering is safer, quicker and more hygienic than bathing.
- Thermostatic showers are essential to avoid scalding.
- Moving and handling risks can be minimised by using suitable equipment.
- Level-access showers cater for all mobility requirements.

PART 5

Supporting individuals in dressing

CHAPTER 13

Keeping up appearances: helping residents to dress

As children, we learn many practical skills, such as walking and talking, but dressing ourselves is one of the last personal care skills that a child gains independence in. Most children master dressing by the age of 5 years, but after this age many children still require assistance with intricacies, such as fastenings.

Dressing and undressing are activities that most of us take for granted and consider being routine. When we are ill, or where there is confusion of thought, dressing can be a tiring and complicated experience. The skills required to undertake personal care activities are very complex. Dressing is one of the most difficult tasks to achieve. Interestingly, with the onset of old age, dressing is one of the first activities to cause problems as people develop physical or cognitive problems.

The function of clothes

Clothing, at its basic level, has a physiological function. It keeps us warm or shields us from basic elements, such as the sun, wind or rain. Materials have been developed and refined to withstand water, high temperatures and even gravitational pressure. This enables human beings to work in extreme situations that would otherwise be impossible.

Anderson (2005) describes 'smart' clothing that contains tiny sensors to gather information about the user and his or her surroundings. At present, the application of smart clothing seems to be aimed at 'extreme sports' and military personnel, but one day they will be commonly available. Some applications of smart clothing are:

- Jackets with battery-powered lighting that is activated at dusk.
- A thermogenerator that monitors and adjusts body temperature.
- Monitoring of blood pressure and insulin levels using 'telecare medicine'.

However, clothing is about more than dealing with the elements and mastering our physical environment; clothing makes a personal statement and has social significance.

Most people give dressing little thought – more care is given to the choice of clothing, rather than the act of dressing itself. Whatever the need or desire for clothing, most people gain some form of satisfaction when feeling well dressed. For years, youths have used clothes to represent their distinctiveness and separateness from adults, yet their attire has become like a uniform, for example Teddy Boys, Mods and Rockers, Punks and Goths. In adulthood, the distinctiveness of clothing may be less stark, but it remains. People alter their appearance with accessories, hairstyles, makeup, cosmetics and skin markings (e.g. piercings and tattoos) to add to the social and cultural message of clothing. Staff wear uniforms to identify staff groups and to differentiate between grades of staff, including within care settings.

Within a care setting

In assessing individuals' need for help, it is important to observe their skills and problem areas before intervening. It is often easier, and tempting, to help slightly, but this can be counterproductive as it can increase dependency, with individuals rapidly relying on others to take total control of the whole process. This may functionally be more efficient for managing the home and staff hours, but it does not enhance independence. Providing assistance can remove the essential value that older people may have placed on their sense of self and belonging.

Helping a person to dress may be frustrating and time-consuming, but by applying some simple techniques or providing small assistive equipment, the core values of the care home are more likely to be achieved. Different techniques and approaches can help individual residents to maintain a maximum level of independence with dressing and undressing and to continue to experience the sense of dressing well. People who have problems with dressing and fastenings may require help with toileting because they are unable to manage their clothing. If suitable clothing is provided they may be able to manage this activity.

Coping with physical impairments

From a physical aspect, dressing requires a good range of movement, balance, coordination, dexterity and grip. Clothes have to be identified as individual garments and items have to be put on in the right sequence and 'straightened up'. The basic starting point is to recognise that taking clothes off is easier than

Table 13.1 An activity to try: dressing.

Imagine that the physical aspect of dressing is difficult because of hemiparesis (partial loss of function down one side of the body due to brain damage).

- Next time you are getting undressed and dressed try to put yourself in that scenario. Analyse where the problems lie.
- How did you manage cuff fastenings and the top buttons or back fastenings of clothing?
- Can you fasten a tie?

putting them on. It doesn't matter how clothes are taken off as long as they eventually come off.

To help with adjustment of clothing and grooming, mirrors should be viewable from a seated and standing position. However, people with cognitive or perceptual difficulties can find mirrors confusing and distracting. Often, it is only by simulating activities (Table 13.1) that we find solutions for others.

■ Using different techniques

Some items, such as a cardigan or fleece, can be removed more easily if they remain fastened and are pulled over the head. Knees can be used to grip the item before removing the last arm from the garment. When putting on a shirt, blouse, cardigan, jacket, jumper, T-shirt or vest, place the 'affected' arm in the garment first, then pull the garment up above the elbow to the armpit before inserting the other arm. When undressing remove the affected (right) arm first and then remove the unaffected (left) arm.

■ Fashion and alternative styles

People who need residential care do not lose their desire to retain their own individual style of dress. As people age, the gradual loss of body flexibility means that older people adapt their clothing to compensate for problem areas. Today's fashions provide a variety of clothing that helps dressing become easier but in a subtle, not overt, way. The concept of inclusive design is an area that has been neglected in the fashion industry, yet clothing is a vital factor to a feeling of self-esteem. Clothing can be gradually replaced with looser items, such as jogging suits that avoid intricate fastenings. Examples include:

- Shirts with zippers rather than buttons are useful to cope with dexterity problems.
- Front-fastening bras.
- Looser-fitting clothing with open necklines that are easier to dress with.

- Longer-length skirts and dresses to preserve modesty and camouflage the wearing of a catheter bag, yet not interfere with walking or propulsion of a wheelchair.
- Fashion shoes with Velcro fastenings that avoid the need for two hands and can be used in conjunction with a shoehorn to avoid bending.
- Elastic cuffs instead of traditional button fastenings at cuffs.

■ **Clothing for those with special needs**

Many people don't need such specialist clothing, but may, because of more sensitive skin, need to dress in more natural materials like cotton and silk. The DLF (2006d) fact sheet recommends clothing for sensitive skins. To reduce moving and handling, clothing may eventually be required for physically dependent people that can be put on from a seated or lying down position. Some residents may need more specialist or customised clothing. For example:

- Wheelchair users can wear garments with a higher waistband at the rear.
- Wider trouser legs will accommodate a catheter bag. Coats and jackets should be short at the back so they are not sat upon if pressure-relieving cushions are used.
- Double-ended zips can be opened to the waist to prevent the zip from curling up.
- Absorbent scarves help with drooling problems.
- Back-opening jackets are easier to manage for people with high dependency needs, e.g. high-level spinal cord lesions.
- Open-backed garments that overlap at the back can help with toileting, yet ensure dignity.
- Some trousers and underpants have extra room to cope with sanitary requirements.

Some common problem areas and suggestions on solutions are provided in Table 13.2.

■ **Locating clothing**

Finding clothing can be facilitated in several ways:

- Ensure belongings are put in familiar places, particularly if personal furniture is brought into the home. Label furniture if needed.
- Encourage residents to select their own clothing or provide just a few choices for them.
- Try arranging the wardrobe so that items are colour-coded.
- De-clutter and remove clothes that are not in season and store in out-of-reach places.

Table 13.2 Some dressing problems, causes and solutions.

Problem	Some causes	Solutions
Impaired hand function causing problems with buttons and zips	Rheumatoid arthritis Strokes Multiple sclerosis Parkinsonism	Buttonhook (a metal loop that is pushed through the button hole and round the button) Use bigger buttons Use Velcro or a loop on a zip Shirts with Velcro fastenings Avoid cuff fastenings – use elasticised wrists and waistbands or jogging suits
Restricted movement in shoulders	Frozen shoulder Arthritis in shoulders	Use dressing stick Choose front-opening cardigans or fleeces rather than jumpers
Difficulty reaching down	Upper or lower limb problems or back pain	Long-handled reachers Store essential items within reach
Difficulty reaching feet	Back or hip or knee problems	Encourage to dress whilst seated on the bed or chair Supply a footstool Pick up stick Stocking gutter or tights aid Sock aid Long-handled shoehorn
Problem tying shoelaces	Loss of hand function in one arm	Teach one-handed method Use elastic laces or coiled laces Shoes with Velcro or elasticised fastenings
Problem tying shoelaces	Back or hip or knee problems	Slip-on shoes and long-handled shoehorn
Unable to see	Visual problems	Ensure lighting is sufficient without glaring Colour code and organise wardrobe so that garments are easier to identify Ensure a label is on the inside back of the garment to enable the back to be located Put clothing away in the correct draw and pair socks
Generalised weakness	Frailty Fatigue Multiple sclerosis	Wear layers of clothing rather than one heavy item (vest/T-shirt, blouse/shirt and fleece Dress in stages, e.g. rest after grooming the dress Lay items out the previous night

- Perhaps lay out clothes in the evening for the following day, or hang them outside the wardrobe.
- Items that the resident needs to access should be within reach.

– Sliding doors are easier to access. They do not require a resident to move backwards with a walking appliance when opening a door.

Good housekeeping issues

The design of the physical environment can either be conducive to dressing, or can add further barriers. When adapting accommodation or building purpose-built extensions, it is essential to look at interior design and environmental aspects. Inclusive design is discussed in Chapter 4; this section concentrates on aspects of the environment that can assist or hinder dressing.

■ Interior design

Lighting and choice of colour are as important as the physical layout and the placing of facilities like electric switches. Lighting should be suitable for the resident, and also for the task. Areas should be illuminated, but there should not be glare. Adequate lighting is important in bedrooms and in wardrobe areas to aid residents with any visual impairment or dementia. Ideally, enable residents to locate a handrail or a light switch; contrasting colour should be used. This concept can be applied to dressing; it is easier to find an item if it is on a contrasting bedspread, particularly if a resident has cognitive or perceptual problems.

■ Environmental aspects

CSCI reports provide details of individual homes and their room spaces based upon the National Minimum Standards (Department of Health, 2003b). Although wheelchair users' rooms should be a minimum of 12 m², and other residents should have a minimum of 10 m² room space, other factors must be taken into consideration:

– There must be sufficient room to manoeuvre a walking appliance or a wheelchair so that access can be gained to all storage areas.
– If residents sit to dress, check that the chair or bed is the right height. The thighs should be parallel to the floor, with the knees at 90°. Chairs with arms are more suitable as they provide assistance to stand, or semi-stand, to pull items up.
– A bed rail or a strategically placed handrail may be needed, either to assist with standing, or to assist when balancing and straightening items.
– Check that the room temperature is correct for the resident.

Conclusion

Although residents of care homes often have multiple problems, it is important to maintain their ability to dress and undress themselves for as long as possible. Apart from the obvious benefits of maintaining privacy and dignity, and retaining maximum range of movement and general physical abilities, it also has a social impact. It enhances self-esteem, and clothing is an expression of individuality within a group context.

It is an essential role of a care assistant to help residents to maintain their appearance by encouraging independence. Ideally, the minimum of assistance should be given. New techniques or alteration to the environment should be made to maximise a person's level of function and to encourage self-motivation.

The application of advances in technical textiles, micro-technologies and new manufacturing techniques will hopefully produce a new era of clothing that has inclusive design.

Key points

- Independence in dressing maintains a resident's privacy and dignity.
- Introduce an alternative technique or an assistive device if a resident has difficulty with dressing.
- Provide advice on more suitable easy-to-manage clothing.
- Ensure the environment is conducive to the dressing process.
- Developments of 'smart' fabrics will enable automatic monitoring of residents' medical conditions.

CHAPTER 14

When it's hard to dress: managing cognitive problems

To dress there has to be an awareness of the need to dress or to change clothes, particularly if they are dirty or soiled. Items have to be found and recognised. There has to be an understanding of which items go on what parts of the body. If more than one item is worn there is a sequence of dressing that needs to be followed. Changing clothing therefore relies on more than the ability to insert limbs into garments and manage fastenings. Dressing requires a high level of cognitive ability, and for some residents these abilities are gradually being eroded because of, for example, dementia causing cognitive problems.

Cognitive problems

Cognition is defined as 'the mental act or process by which knowledge is acquired, including perception, intuition and reasoning' (Collins, 2004). Cognitive problems can result from a loss of one or more processes involving higher intellectual functioning, perception, reasoning and intuition. Residents of care homes often have multiple cognitive problems that can make the act of changing clothes an overwhelming experience.

Cognitive problems superimposed on physical difficulties can cause both physical problems coping with garments, and an inability to put clothes on in the correct sequence. Cognitive problems are complex, but it is not necessary to understand exactly why a person has those problems – it is more important to be aware of how to help to overcome difficulties. Murphy (2000) says:

> If you stop to consider the complexity of movement that is orchestrated by the brain to do something as simple as bend the arm in just the right way to facilitate getting it into the sleeve of a shirt, you begin to understand how impossible the most simple movements become when the brain can no longer locate or send the signals that make that arm work at will.

When a resident is getting dressed, consider the following questions:

- Does the resident know why he/she is getting dressed?
- Is the resident reluctant to dress?
- Is the resident reluctant to change clothes in front of someone?
- Can the resident find his/her clothing?
- Can the resident put items on in the right sequence?
- Are there any problems with perception?

Does the resident know why he/she is getting dressed?

Residents who have memory problems or early signs of dementia can be disorientated in time and place. It is important to establish a routine. It is helpful to have clocks with the right time and a large dial or digital numbers sited in a prominent place. The time of day can also be reinforced by subtly introducing it into conversation. Similarly reinforcement of location is important. Staff can make reference to the place a resident is in subtle ways, for example 'you have made your bedroom look good'. These prompts help orientate an individual, and thereby help them recognise that they are about to get dressed.

Is the resident reluctant to dress?

If there is a recent loss of interest in dressing, or doing other activities, then it is important to check to see whether or not there is a physical, cognitive or psychological problem; for example medication, loss of dexterity or depression. If residents are unwilling to change clothing, then try different tactics. For example, encourage them to change clothing after they bathe or shower, before they go out, or before a visitor comes. They may have favourite items of clothing that they like wearing, so arrange for several of these items to be purchased so that, after a bath, the 'same outfit' can be worn again. Try to find out how frequently they changed clothing before admission. Provided the clothes do not smell or are not soiled there is no reason why the same clothing can't be worn the next day. Being told to change your clothing can be very embarrassing, so deal with this tactfully. Often, residents may have some difficulty choosing the proper clothing to wear. Rather than overwhelm them with choice, at each stage of dressing only provide a few items to choose from.

Is the resident reluctant to change clothes in front of someone?

For most people, changing clothing is a private experience. Perhaps residents have only recently needed help, and may therefore feel embarrassed. Use this opportunity to get to know the resident, and try to allow him or her to do as much as possible.

> Having other people's hands and eyes on our naked, not-so-beautiful body is an acutely uncomfortable experience... it is an admission that this person is no longer able to manage for himself, that he has in fact become like a child who must have help and be told when to dress. (Mace and Rabins, 1999)

It is important to bear in mind that reluctance may be more than expected embarrassment, and may be as a result of a problem that is deeper seated.

Can the resident find his/her clothing?

Simplify the environment (Chapter 13) by de-cluttering draws and wardrobes and put items back in the same place each time. If residents can no longer read words, it may help to put pictures on drawers; even if this is unsightly it will assist.

Can the resident put items on in the right sequence?

Try laying all items out in the correct sequence, with underwear on top. The resident does not in this case have to engage in more complex thought processes of trying to remember where things are kept, or in which order to get dressed. Reduce the number of layers worn and avoid intricate fastenings. Undressing is far easier than dressing: it does not matter how clothes are taken off, or indeed where they are put.

Are there any problems with perception?

Perceptual problems can arise from many causes, including dementia, head injuries, brain tumours or strokes that have affected the part of the brain that mainly deals with perception. If residents suffer from perceptual problems, identification of items of clothing can be problematic. Clothes may be put on in the wrong order and often on the wrong part of the body. Perceptual problems broadly fall into two categories:

- **Agnosia** (inability to recognise everyday items). Try to make items easy to identify by putting them on contrasting bedspreads, or leave clothing on hangers. Use contrasting colours for garments. Purchase reversible clothing or clothing that has no definite front or back, so it will not matter if the garment is worn back to front or inside out. Many fashion items are constructed in this way.
- **Apraxia** (can recognise and describe an item but cannot perform an action). Try to minimise the layers worn, pick simple clothing and avoid fastenings.

Helping a resident with cognition problems involves focusing on making the process of dressing easier. Often, by observing behaviour, blockages can be identified and methods discovered to overcome problems. Once skills are lost, it may not be possible to regain them – but by care staff adopting a positive coordinated approach and teaching new techniques, a resident can be helped to achieve as much as possible. Table 14.1 offers some useful solutions for common dressing problems.

General hints

Use 'backward chaining' techniques and simplify the process by using a minimum number of items. Verbally encourage and help the resident to identify the garments. Perhaps start by encouraging residents to take nightwear off and providing assistance with daywear. Concentrate on garments with similar 'take off/put on' techniques, such as vests/T-shirts and cardigans/shirts. Provide assistance only if needed. Gradually decrease the amount of support provided until the resident's optimum level is reached. It is important to work in partnership with any visiting therapist to help overcome problem areas:

Table 14.1 Examples of problems with dressing and suggested solutions.

Behaviour	Suggestions
Dressing inappropriately	Provided the clothing is right for the season, and is not offensive to others, it should not matter what they choose to wear
Unable to recognise an item if held the wrong way up (form constancy problems)	Items can be placed on hangers rather than laid on the bed or care staff can hold it up in the correct way as part of helping a person decide what to wear
Problems differentiating individual items if several are on a bed	Stay in the room and put one item on the bed at a time. Use a contrasting or plain bedspread
Difficulty finding an item due to loss of visual field, for example hemianopia	Place items within their range of vision
Neglecting to dress one side of the body due to failure to recognise a limb as being their own (anosognosia)	Dress in front of a long mirror and gradually encourage more movement towards the neglected side
Putting clothes on upside down, inside out or in the wrong order Putting items on the wrong part of their body or in a disorganised manner	Initially buy garments with easy to identify fronts and backs, e.g. V-neck or round or polo necks Simplify the dressing process so that garments require similar techniques, e.g. T-shirt and jumper Buy reversible clothing Put labels on the back of a garment but remove labels when a person can no longer help to dress as these can irritate and may lead to constant undressing
Putting items on in the wrong order	Place garments within reach either on the bed or a chair in a 'put-on' order
Problems coordinating movements when grasping garments (visuo-spatial problems)	Place near to resident Avoid intricate fastenings
Keep getting undressed	Try to ascertain why they want to undress. They may lose social controls and feel uncomfortable in clothing for some reason: Are they too hot? Perhaps they need to remove an outer layer of clothing. Are the clothes comfortable to wear? Do they need the toilet? Are they looking for something to do? Do they think it is time for bed? Are they tired and want to have a rest on the bed?
Short attention span	Provide gentle prompts and pass the next item to the resident using clear simple phrases, not long complex sentences

- Leave residents to do as much as they can for themselves.
- Provide gentle, clear prompts and reminders to correct the sequence of dressing.
- Talk about the next item of clothing in short phrases, not long complicated sentences.
- Try an easier technique – for example, encourage residents to sit while dressing, to use a footstool and to put the garment on with any weaker limb in first.
- Simplify the process – for example, fold a sock down to aid foot insertion.
- Break the task of dressing into simple stages. Provide praise when a stage is successfully completed.
- Allow plenty of time.
- Pay attention to footwear, ensuring it gives adequate support and the shoes have slip-resistant soles.
- Provide subtle help by giving physical help without drawing attention to the resident's problems.

Murphy (2000) gives a good example of supporting helping:

Tom was still able to get the belt into the front loops of his trousers by himself, but always missed the back loops. By hovering behind him I was able to slip the belt into the back loops, facilitating this part of his dressing routine without being too obvious. When he lost the ability to buckle the belt, I reached around him and buckled it for him. By working behind him he was less aware of the amount of help he was actually receiving.

Conclusion

It is an essential part of the role of a care assistant to help residents to maintain their appearance. This affords them dignity and self-respect. Where possible, staff should aim to encourage total independence in dressing, but in some circumstances this may not be possible. Instead, the minimum level of assistance should be aimed for and techniques adopted to maximise a person's level of function. In the early stages this may actually take more time than doing things for individuals, but in terms of the positive care experience that it provides it is much more satisfying for residents and staff alike.

Key points

■ Identify where the problem is when a resident is dressing.
■ Looking good is critical to self-esteem and well-being.
■ Provide clear prompts using gestures and short phrases.
■ Try to simplify the process of dressing by reducing layers and avoiding complex fastenings.

PART 6

Helping individuals to eat and drink

CHAPTER 15

Food for thought: providing solutions to feeding problems

For most people, eating is a pleasurable experience; often associated with cultural and religious significance. As people age, or develop physical and cognitive problems, the consumption of healthy food can be a challenge. Less saliva is produced, and tooth loss and denture problems add to mastication difficulties. Senses often diminish with age, making food smell or taste different.

Healthy eating: implications for care homes

Food should contain adequate vitamins, minerals and calories, particularly when special diets are required. Good nutrition is essential; a whole science and industry has developed in relation to this. Smith (2004a) explains how dieticians can help with nutritional requirements and facilitate changes to practice within care homes. A special social event can be made, for example: a pea and pie supper, a fish and chip night, a curry evening or a Yorkshire afternoon tea – accompanied by music to make it a themed event. Care homes should ensure that meal times are enjoyable experiences and not just a perfunctory task to be undertaken.

Before eating

Some residents may prefer either to eat alone in their rooms or to be part of a smaller group setting. They may have special religious or cultural requirements. Different cultures have distinct approaches to the way food is shared and eaten, or even worshipped or tabooed. Staff should be aware of cultural rituals or family habits, ensuring that these are maintained in a care home setting. For example:

- Food etiquette – utensils, place settings, meal times and type of food consumed.
- Rituals used before meals and offering blessing of food or grace.
- Religious rites.
- A prohibition during preparation of food or before a meal begins, including the type of food eaten.

Establishing these preferences should be part of the assessment process and needs should be identified and remembered when planning meal times. Table 15.1 provides some examples of general feeding problems and solutions.

Assisting a resident

Residents should be encouraged to be as independent as possible by adopting different techniques, or by using assistive devices. If they are unable to cut food up with assistive devices, then cut the food before taking it to the table or provide food that does not require cutting. Offer help in a discreet way.

Individual residents may have particular needs and may require assistance with feeding. If residents are unable to manage adapted cutlery and require feeding, this activity should be carried out with patience and sensitivity. Feeding someone can be enjoyable or a chore to get over quickly, depending on how it is approached by the individuals concerned. Throughout the meal the resident should be engaged in conversation, as much as is possible, and encouraged to eat slowly, at his or her own pace, with regular sips of drink provided. Ideally, the carer should be seated in front of the person he/she is feeding or within his/her clear field of vision. Don't perch on the side of the resident's chair or carry out conversations with other people, or feed two residents at once. Table 15.2 lists some practical and cognitive problems that residents may experience and offers some solutions.

Seating and positioning

The right ambiance can be created by attractive and pleasant surroundings if attention is paid to the dining environment and appropriate lighting. Correct seating and posture are vital.

Table 15.1 General feeding problems.

Problem	Alternatives
Eating takes a long time	■ Smaller, more frequent portions with refills (less daunting and food won't get cold) ■ Provide high-calorie snacks and nutritional drinks between meals
Chewing or swallowing foods	■ Check that dentures fit properly ■ Try different replacement foods, e.g. Replace fruit with fruit juices, soft canned or pureed fruits Replace raw vegetables with soups, juices, creamed and mashed cooked vegetables Replace meat with minced meats or high-protein food, e.g. dairy produce Replace bread with soft cereals, rice and soft cakes ■ Encourage smaller mouthfuls to avoid 'squirreling food' in the cheeks ■ Provide easy to digest food that requires little chewing and avoid: Food with 'skins' that can stick to the palate, e.g. tomato Small, coarse and hard foods, e.g. peanuts, potato crisps and hard toast, as these can be accidentally inhaled Sharp food: take meat off the bone and buy filleted fish Shredded vegetables, e.g. coleslaw, carrots and lettuce Acidic, spicy foods that can irritate the throat Mixtures of food textures (confusing to the mouth, can cause choking) Water (can cause choking); try using chilled water or thicken liquids
Poor appetite	■ Check medication (may affect appetite) ■ Check for mouth sores or ulcers ■ Improve the flavour and appearance of the food ■ Provide favourite foods to tempt the appetite ■ Check for anxiety or depression (can affect appetite) ■ Postpone eating if residents are tired or upset. Restart when convenient ■ Eat higher-calorie meals 'little and often', e.g. dairy produce, oils, nuts, carbohydrate and protein supplements. Add dry milk powder to foods with sauces ■ Drink high-nutrient liquids such as juice or milk, instead of coffee, tea or sodas ■ Make meal time pleasurable ■ Perhaps move to another table ■ Encourage light exercise to stimulate appetite
Changes in taste	■ Eat flavoured or spicier foods ■ Drink liquids with meals to rinse away any unpleasant taste ■ Add sauces, stuffings and side dishes to foods ■ Use plastic utensils if a metallic taste sensation occurs ■ Avoid foods that taste unpleasant

Table 15.1 (*continued*)

Problem	Alternatives
Constipation	■ Refer to GP and find out the cause. Causes include: Insufficient exercise (can impair gastrointestinal function) Insufficient fluid intake (2–3 litres or 6 to 8 glasses a day) Lack of dietary fibre (increase intake of fruit, vegetables, wholemeal cereals, prunes and add natural bran to foods in puddings, stews and soups) ■ Hot lemon water helps stimulate the bowel
Problems taking medication	■ Try alternative form of medication (sugar-coated capsules, crush tablets and place in food, liquid) ■ Seek advice from pharmacist
Fatigue	■ Provide smaller more frequent meals (eating involves several muscles and requires oxygen, often increasing shortness of breath) ■ Full stomach can press on the diaphragm, restricting lung capacity ■ Provide a short rest before eating

■ Table height
The table height should allow forearms to be rested on the tabletop.

■ Chairs
The chair should encourage a good sitting posture. Full-length armrests provide support when rising and sitting, but they can prevent close access to the table and desk-type chair arms may be better. Fabric upholstered chairs, although more comfortable and attractive than a vinyl chair, are difficult to clean. A wooden 'ski' base will make pushing an occupied chair away from the table easier.

- Place the resident's feet on the floor or on a footstool, with ankles, hips and knees at right angles. Seat him/her upright, then ask him/her to lean slightly forward with shoulders relaxed (not hunched).
- Ensure that the sitting position facilitates the feeding process.
- Specialised seating to provide postural support to the resident to facilitate eating and digestion may be required.
- Position the chair so that residents who are prone to choking are easily accessible.

■ Feeding position
During feeding, residents' heads should be kept slightly down and forward. If the head is back, the risk of gagging or choking increases. Stabilise unsteady heads by placing your palm on the resident's forehead or behind the neck, or provide support with a head or neck rest. Residents who are bed-bound should

Table 15.2 Some practical and cognitive feeding problems and solutions.

Problems	Solutions
Spillage of food when feeding, causing seepage onto clothing	Feeding bib or apron
Tremor	Weighted cutlery, cups and heavier plates Swivel cutlery and deep-bowl spoons Plastic cutlery (prevents dental damage) Unbreakable crockery
Upper limb weakness	Lightweight cups and cutlery Long-handled or angled cutlery Mobile arm supports and feeding systems
One-handed use	Scoop bowls and plate guards Sloping curved sided plates or straight-sided 'pasta' type dishes Partitioned plates and bowls Plates on suckers or on non-slip material Rocker knife or cheese knife Cutlery to cope with one-handed use, for example a rounded blade with a fork at the end; a fork with one spear thickened and sharpened to provide a cutting edge; a fork, spoon and knife combined ('splayd'); a fork with a cutting roller on the underside. Provide no-cut food (for example, casseroles) or pre-cut chunks
Slowness, causing food to cool	Pre-heated hot plate Bowl with sealed hot water container beneath Insulated bowls and plates to keep food warm (some have a hollow base that can be filled with hot water to keep the food warm) Insulated cup or cups with narrowing tops
Poor grip	Enlarged or moulded handles on cutlery Cups with two handles
Limited or no grip	Hand strap with palm pocket for cutlery
Difficultly managing cup	Fill half full, use lightweight cup or cup with spout Enlarged handle/double-handled cup Add handle with 'Gripkit' (mouldable compound) Sports' drink containers (more aesthetic than feeding beakers)
Sensation impaired	Insulated cups
Tendency to spill drink	Anti-spill cup (wider or weighted base) Cups with two handles
Restricted neck bending	Angled cup Cup with cut out at back
Unable to lift cup to mouth	Flexible/wide straws (thicker substances) Bulldog clip (pass straw through it to secure) Straws with one-way valves
Problems controlling liquid flow	Larger spout Vacuum cup with valve in lid

Table 15.2 (*continued*)

Problems	Solutions
Difficulty drinking	Clip-on straws with a one-way valve
Crockery moving during eating	Remove tablecloth and use non-slip mat or non-slip matting Heavier plates
Speech problems	Word cards or picture cards to facilitate choice/preference
Visual problems	Utensils that contrast with table or cloth Bright patterned glasses Partitioned plates and bowls

not be given fluids, solids or medications when in a supine position. A sitting position should be adopted, with the head of the bed elevated to a 45–90° angle by adjusting the bed, by placing three or more pillows behind the shoulder and neck, or by using a foam wedge.

Crockery and cutlery

Many residents have difficulty with feeding as a result of both physical and cognitive problems. Appropriate feeding utensils and condiments should be provided within easy reach of the resident, and within their range of vision. If eyesight is poor, then guide the resident to what is on the plate by relating food position to a clock face, for example: meat at 6 o'clock, vegetables at 10 o'clock.

Non-slip mats or non-slip netting have a multitude of uses, including giving crockery more stability. Non-slip materials can be placed direct onto the table surface, but many homes like to use tablecloths to give a 'homely feel'. Non-slip mats will work on tablecloths, but the cloth itself can slip on the table.

Meeting individual needs

Appropriate feeding equipment can help overcome physical problems and help achieve a resident's independence. Local integrated community equipment stores (ICES) and occupational therapists can offer advice on suitable equipment. When choosing feeding equipment, bear in mind:

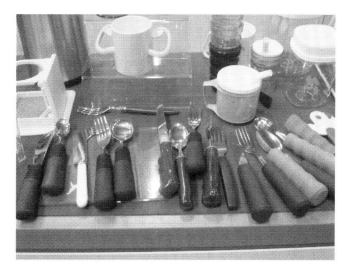

Examples of feeding aids (© Julie Swann 2007).

- Is the equipment simple to assemble?
- Are the parts difficult to clean?
- Can cutlery and crockery items be washed in a dishwasher?
- Is the item strong and durable?
- How many spare items will you need?
- Are residents safe when using sharp items?

Difficulty swallowing

Ensure food goes 'down the right tube' – the oesophagus, not the trachea – otherwise choking and aspiration pneumonia can follow. If residents are unable to take food by mouth there are several other methods available using the gastrointestinal tract for the delivery of nutrients, including food and oral supplements. Enteral feeding (EFT) is needed if a resident is unable to eat or to tolerate enough food and/or oral supplements to meet his or her nutritional needs. Dysphagia (difficulty swallowing) is the most common primary reason for initiating ETF or aiming to improve or maintain nutritional status, malabsorption and anorexia. Summersall and Wight (2004) outline how a speech and language therapist can assist with swallowing problems in dementia. Collier (2004) describes the main methods of enteral feeding as being:

- **Pump feeding**: An electronic feeding pump delivers feed at a set rate per hour over a pre-set dose/time period.

- **Bolus feeding**: Feed is administered into the feeding tube via a syringe.
- **Gravity feeding**: This rarely used method involves the feedbag attached to the enteral feeding tube and feed drips in via gravity.

The common routes for ETF (tube feeding) are:

- **Nasogastric tubes**

A tube is inserted through a nostril, down the throat and into the stomach. This is temporary, but can be pulled out accidentally.

- **Pericutaneous endoscopic gastrostomy (PEG)**

A tube is inserted via the abdomen into the stomach and is usually for long-term use. Residents can receive tube feedings and an oral diet, so even if the oral quantities are not nutritionally significant, psychological benefits are gained. A 'button' tube has a very short tube attached to the stomach with a longer 'snap-on' tube for use during feedings. A plastic cap covers the opening when not in use.

- **Jejunostomy tube (J-tube)**

The tube is implanted below the stomach, directly into the small intestine. This reduces the risk that formula will reflux into the oesophagus, the trachea and the lungs and cause aspiration. Disadvantages are likelihood of diarrhoea and increased probability of the very narrow tube getting clogged.

Dementia and perceptual problems

Residents with dementia can become increasingly difficult to persuade to eat, particularly if they are agitated. Regular meal times will help to establish routines, and several smaller courses will be more suitable than one main meal. Try to reduce distractions; for example, turn off the TV, 'de-clutter' the table and place condiments, napkin and drink in the correct place.

Encourage eating by making food look more appetising by using contrasting colours and different food textures. Avoid patterned plates and use plain ones that contrast with food on the plate. Social etiquette is important to maintain. Provide suitable eating implements (spoons are easier than forks, straight-sided pasta bowls are easier than plates). If residents refuse to use cutlery, or can't manage cutlery, cut food into manageable mouthfuls or provide finger food, and allow longer times for consuming meals.

Conclusion

Eating is part of a social experience and it is possible, with a little imagination, to help facilitate social interaction. Food should be nutritious, tasty and attractive. If residents experience problems with eating, there are a range of different techniques and devices that can make meal times pleasurable and positive social experiences, whilst maintaining their independence for as long as possible.

Key points

- Food should be nutritious, tasty and attractive.
- Maintain cultural rituals and social habits.
- Create attractive and pleasant dining surroundings.
- Seating and table height should facilitate eating.
- Ensure appropriate feeding equipment is provided.
- Specialist feeding systems are available if residents are unable to take food orally.

Continence management

CHAPTER 16

Supporting individuals to go to the toilet

For most people, going to the toilet is a natural, everyday activity that is taken for granted. As people age or develop physical problems, rising from the toilet, cleansing and managing clothing can become increasingly difficulty. However, with thought and relatively minor adaptations, individuals can be assisted to use the toilet.

Care homes generally have well-equipped bathrooms and toilets. Outside of the care home, amenities offered by retail premises such as large department stores, shopping centres or cafés often have an absence of suitable toilet facilities. This chapter concentrates on two main aspects: cultural and practical considerations.

Cultural considerations

It is important to be aware of a resident's cultural and religious requirements. Some cultures place a very high emphasis on cleanliness, in both physical and spiritual aspects, and prescriptive routines must be followed. For example: the Khalifah Project (2004) notes that Muslims must 'enter the toilet with the left foot and leave with the right foot'. It is considered 'detestable' to stand while urinating. After using the toilet, purification of the peritoneal area by running water ('Istinja') is required. Therefore, to comply with some religious beliefs, bidets or basins should be provided in each toilet to enable people to wash themselves with running water. Dependent patients may appreciate having a jug of warm water poured over their peritoneal area before being taken off the commode, bedpan or toilet.

Practical considerations

People with disabilities, or with increasing frailty, may experience mild to substantial problems with personal care activities that are added to by design problems. When designing accessible areas, particularly in care homes, ODPM (2006) provides useful guidance and should be followed for all new property. These regulations take into consideration the needs of people with visual or hearing impairments, people with learning difficulties and people whose lack of tactile sensitivity can cause them to be injured by touching hot or sharp surfaces.

Sometimes access to the toilet area may be adequate; but if a toilet door opens inwards, this reduces the space. In a small cubicle it is difficult to close the door. For people encumbered by children, shopping bags or luggage, this often requires the occupant to move to the side to when closing and opening the door. People using walking aids or a wheelchair and those who need assistance may not be able to gain access without leaving the door open. This can be a very humiliating experience. With foresight, most cubicles could easily have been made longer.

ODPM (2006) recognises that:

> the provision of an enlarged cubicle in a separate-sex toilet washroom can be of benefit to ambulant disabled people, as well as parents with children, and people (e.g. those with luggage) who need an enlarged space.

The Building Regulations (2000) stated that all toilet doors on new property with public access should open outwards. Outward-opening doors provide greater access in an emergency; for example if a person has had a fall in the cubicle.

When designing products and buildings, average limb lengths, height and range of movement (anthropometrics) are used. Vital general factors in connection with personal care activities include the following.

■ Visual contrast

Part of the Building Regulations for public buildings requires that, 'the surface finish of sanitary fittings and grab bars contrasts visually with background wall and floor finishes, and there is also visual contrast between wall and floor finishes'. Several companies retail toilets, washbasins and handrails that comply with the regulations, with contrasting handrails. Decorating the toilet walls in a contrasting colour to the handrail, basin and toilet will help people who are visually impaired, as will the supply of coloured toilet paper and coloured disinfectant in the cistern to colour the toilet water. By placing items so that they can be easily seen and within reach, tasks can be more easily achieved. Clearing the area from clutter provides the minimum of distraction to enable the task to be concentrated upon.

■ Doors and internal space

Doors that contrast with the wall colour are easier to locate. Door handles should contrast with the door and usable with a closed fist (ODPM, 2006), for example automatic opening or lever handles. Doors should open easily (with less than 20 N (newton) force). A horizontal closing bar fixed to the inside face makes closure easier for a wheelchair user.

■ Locks

Locks should be operable using one hand and by people with limited dexterity; for example, light-action privacy bolts (ODPM, 2006). In an emergency, doors should have a release mechanism capable of being opened from the outside (ODPM, 2006). Some of the new locks in public toilets have chunky grips, but can be difficult to turn – a simple latch mechanism is easier.

■ Emergency pull cords

Pull cords for emergency alarms should have intact 50 mm bangles at two levels: one at 800–1000 mm and the other at 100 mm from the floor (ODPM, 2006); i.e. reachable from the floor if a fall occurs, and reachable from the toilet so that assistance can be summoned. Often emergency pull cords are broken or tied up out of reach, or the bangles are broken. The cords should be red, not white, as this prevents residents mistaking alarm cords for light pulls. To prevent accidental triggering, cords should not be placed near a handrail or toilet paper dispenser.

■ Lighting

Appropriate levels of lighting are important, especially when an older person's sight has deteriorated. Lighting should be appropriate for the task, and of adequate luminosity. Switches with large push pads should be used in preference to pull cords, as these and automatic lighting are easier to use.

■ Mirrors

A common mistake is to have several rows of tiling sited above the sink and the mirror placed above. This will exclude those who use wheelchairs. Mirror tiles could be used instead, or a tilt mirror or mirror on an extendable arm installed.

■ Towel rails and dispensers

Towels or hand dryers should be positioned within reach of wheelchair users and ambulant residents, and should be reachable from the toilet.

■ Accessing public toilets

For many people with mobility difficulties, accessing and using toilets away from home can be a stressful and difficult experience. Fortunately, most towns have an accessible toilet that is operated by a key obtained from RADAR (http://www.radar.org.uk/), tourist offices and some local authorities. The whereabouts of all National Key Scheme (NKS) toilets are listed in RADAR's (2005) NKS Guide, a useful publication to help locate accessible toilets for trips out with residents.

Toilets

Toilets should be around 480 cm (19 in) high (ODPM, 2006); therefore, some may need raising by a toilet seat, frame or combined seat and frame. Many toilet frames are adjustable in height and width. These should be adjusted to individual needs if the frame is to be used solely by one person. For frames in communal areas they should be adjusted to a generous width allowing for residents with larger hip widths. For bariatric (overweight) residents, a combined toilet seat and frame or a commode over the toilet is useful. These can take their weight, avoiding any damage to the toilet. Contoured seats are comfortable and supportive. There are several padded or inflatable wipe-down seats that are useful for frail or thin people.

If there is weakness in one side of the body the individual's weight will not be placed equally on the toilet frame and it can tip. However, floor fixing kits are available for some free standing frames.

Toilet rails

Wall rails can help individuals to stand up or transfer or to provide stability when males are urinating. Rails can be used to help maintain a sitting posture or standing balance when assistance is provided to manage clothing. Drop-down rails can help, but must be firmly attached to a wall. Rails should be sited within reach. Many toilets have rails that are in the wrong place. The optimum position to assist with rising is placement at hip level when standing. ODPM (2006) provides suggested layouts for toilets to facilitate access by ambulant disabled and wheelchair users.

Toilet paper

Toilet paper must be within reach and extractable by one hand (ODPM, 2006). A roll lock or interleaved single-sheet paper will help if limited range of movement prevents extraction using a one-handed method. Contrasting toilet paper helps residents who have visual impairments.

Cleansing

A bidet bowl or an electrically powered 'add-on bidet' can be used on top of a toilet pan to rinse the peritoneal area. Several companies produce toilets that wash and dry the user when seated, e.g. a Clos-o-mat.

Urinals

Many men experience difficulties when coping with the process of toileting due to physical impairments that affect their upper limbs. A reduction in dexterity, swollen arthritic hands or incoordination can adversely affect the process and mechanics of urination. Problems can arise managing clothing fastening and negotiating underwear. Aiming into a toilet bowl can be difficult and lead to urine being spilt on the floor or, embarrassingly, down clothing. Some men may urinate in inappropriate places, for example waste paper bins and sinks. It is easier to do this than to attempt to stand or sit at the toilet. The provision of a urinal can help and the use of urinals is being piloted in some care homes. Many urinals are available, including sensoroperated urinals that flush after usage.

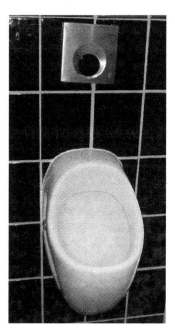

Sensor operated male urinal (© Julie Swann 2007).

Hand washing

Lever taps or sensor-operated taps are suitable for most hand problems. ODPM (2006) states that, 'the finger rinse basin and other accessories should allow a person to wash and dry hands while seated on the WC'.

There are many assistive devices available to assist with toileting. The Disabled Living Foundation (2006e) fact sheet *Choosing Toilet Equipment and Accessories* outlines some of the available equipment that may be of assistance.

Conclusion

On admission to a care environment, it is important to make no assumptions and to establish individual needs. Toileting is an area of everyday activity that individuals may find embarrassing to talk about, so it is critical for staff to use their initiative. Approaching the subject in an understanding way is the best style.

Within the home, attention needs to be paid to the practical environment by designing the living space to best effect. It is particularly important to ensure that residents' cultural needs are met, and care staff must preserve individuals' dignity.

Key points

- Establish individual needs and make no assumptions.
- Ensure that cultural needs are met during toileting.
- Ensure that residents are able to manage clothing and transfers.
- Adapt *en suites* to individual needs and ensure that all items are in reach.
- Use building regulations as a template for public and communal areas.
- Use visually contrasting materials to aid identification of fixtures.

CHAPTER 17

Urinary continence

NHS Direct (2006a) estimates that 3–6 million people in the UK have some degree of urinary incontinence owing to partial or total loss of bladder control. Urinary incontinence is not necessarily part of the ageing process; there may be medical, physiological or other reasons. Health Press (2005a) states that:

> The idea that it [incontinence] affects only the elderly is completely out of date – the popularity of active sports, such as jogging, has caused more younger women to notice the problem.

However, the occurrence of incontinence does increase with ageing, being twice as common in women than men (NHS Direct, 2006a). Urinary incontinence affects the quality of life for many older people – although many causes are treatable. Incontinence, therefore, is not an inevitable part of ageing. If it develops, medical advice should be sought to eliminate the following underlying medical reasons:

- Is there an infection? If so, antibiotics will alleviate the problem.
- Is medication causing incontinence? Some medication, such as tranquillizers and sedatives, can affect control of the bladder muscles.
- Are drinks acting as a diuretic? Alcohol and caffeine drinks should be reduced and other fluids encouraged; for example, water and cranberry juice, not tea, coffee or cola.
- Is the client obese? Try to encourage exercise and a healthy diet.
- Does the client have weak pelvic floor muscles? If so, pelvic floor exercises will help.
- Is the resident depressed? Medication, or simply listening, may help.

How continence is achieved

During the day and night, the bladder fills automatically. The urge to void can normally be postponed until an appropriate place is found. Basic knowledge of bladder and body mechanics helps us to understand continence problems.

■ **Sphincter and pelvic floor muscles**

If the sphincter or pelvic floor muscle is weak or damaged, then incontinence can occur, particularly if excessive pressure is on the bladder. This is termed 'stress urinary incontinence' (SUI).

■ **Sensors within the bladder**

Sensors inform us when our bladder is full or empty. However, sometimes an urge to urinate can occur when the bladder isn't full, or the bladder may start contracting at the wrong time. This urge urinary incontinence (UUI) is often a result of intrinsic neurological disease.

■ **Nervous system**

When nerves connecting the brain (the micturition centre) and spinal cord are damaged, a mixture of SUI and UUI occurs.

Stress urinary incontinence

The most common type of incontinence is SUI. Newman (2003) notes that 35% of incontinent elderly people have SUI. It can be embarrassing and distressing if a small amount of urine leaks out during physical activity, such as coughing, sneezing, vomiting, bending, lifting and even walking or laughing. This can occur during pregnancy, after childbirth and the menopause or if a person is obese (due to weakness of pelvic floor muscles resulting from an increase in abdominal pressure).

Table 17.1 Bladder re-training drill (adapted from Health Press Ltd, 2005b).

Bladder re-training is based on passing urine by the clock at regular intervals. If 'holding on' is difficult for the resident, distraction techniques may be useful, e.g. watching TV.
Days 1 and 2 Start by choosing an interval that the resident feels fairly confident he/she can achieve, such as 1–2 hours. This should be continued for two days.
Days 3 and 4 The resident should increase the interval between emptying by 15 minutes and continue with this interval for two days.
Day 5 onwards When the resident is comfortable with the extra 15 minutes, he/she should increase it again. As each interval becomes manageable, it can be increased again.

The Continence Foundation (2001) describes the pelvic floor muscle as a large sling (or 'hammock') of muscles stretching across the floor of the pelvis, forming an 'undercarriage'. Bo *et al.* (1999) carried out a six-month trial of different treatments for SUI; namely pelvic floor exercises, electrical stimulation and vaginal cones, comparing these to no treatment. Women doing pelvic floor (Kegal) exercises improved the most. Men with 'leakage problems' after urination also found pelvic floor exercises helpful.

Leaflets on pelvic floor exercises are obtainable from GPs, continence advisors, physiotherapists or the internet – for example, the Continence Foundation web site (`http://www.continence-foundation.org.uk/`). Exercises can be practiced individually with residents, particularly during toileting, and some can be incorporated into a 'movement to music' session.

Urge urinary incontinence

Unstable or overactive bladders may feel 'full', causing the bladder to contract too early or empty completely before a toilet is reached. Urge urinary incontinence (UUI) can be triggered by a sudden change of position. Newman (2003) notes that causes include carcinoma; therefore any asymptomatic haematuria (blood in the urine) requires further evaluation.

Re-training the bladder (Table 17.1) can improve urge incontinence and frequency. By gradually stretching the bladder's capacity, a longer time interval becomes possible, after the perceived 'urge', before the bladder needs to empty. This reduces the likelihood of leaking urine before a toilet is reached.

Medication, for example anticholinergics, relax the bladder by blocking nerve impulses, but may produce side-effects such as dry mouth, blurred vision and constipation.

Check the pattern of frequency of voiding by recording this for a few days. Then gradually extend the time before voiding, aiming for 3–5 hours (5–7 times a day). Often a combination of drugs and bladder retraining works well with UUI.

Other forms of incontinence

- **Nocturia**: when people need to visit the toilet frequently during the night.
- **Reflex bladder**: a loss of bladder control, perhaps developed after injury or illness, such as spinal injuries and multiple sclerosis. Residents may require intermittent or continuous catheterisation.

■ **Overflow incontinence**: rare in women but common in men, as an enlarged prostrate gland can press on the urethra. The area behind the obstruction becomes tense and highly pressurised, causing a regular release of a small involuntary dribble of urine, which initially may occur nocturnally. The bladder cannot fill up or empty completely, leaving a residue of urine in the bladder. The obstruction can be removed by surgery.

Positive practical approaches

Continence and toileting are complex tasks requiring many functions, including: recognising a need to void, motivation, route finding, cognition, mobility, clothing management, voiding and cleansing. Environmental obstacles that may need addressing and other positive steps can be taken to reduce incontinence among residents. Consider the following:

■ **Recognising a resident's need to visit the toilet**
The Alzheimer's Association (2006) web site describes common signs to look for, including restlessness, anxiety, agitation, pacing, unusual sounds, facial expressions, sudden behavioural changes, pulling at clothes, dropping pants and suddenly stopping eating. These signs are particularly important to notice if residents are unable to communicate their needs effectively.

■ **Inappropriate urination**
Look for reasons and adopt an ABC of behaviour (antecedent, behaviour and consequence). If toilet facilities are difficult to use or locate, residents may void in inappropriate places.

It is natural and easier for male residents to stand than to partially undress and transfer onto a toilet to urinate. Male residents may have problems supporting themselves and directing urine flow when standing, and therefore may resort to using a sink. Wall urinals will solve this problem and sensor-operated ones are available. Alternatively a urinal can be kept near the toilet.

■ **Maintaining a routine**
Establish a routine of regularly toileting even after an episode of incontinence, ensuring that the bladder is never over-full. There is a difference between increasing bladder capacity and letting residents sit and hold on until the effort of rising, transferring or walking puts pressure on the bladder and causes voiding.

■ **Assisting with toileting**

Ensure that residents have suitable mobility equipment to enable them to manoeuvre safely. Provide help in a reassuring manner to preserve dignity and modesty. If transferring space is limited, then consider using a wheeled commode chair or a hoist. Give verbal cues and guide appropriately. Provide environmental clues – 'look for the blue door' is an easier verbal clue than, 'the toilet is five doors down the corridor'.

■ **Ability to cleanse self**

Put essential items within reach, noting whether residents have limited dexterity and range of movements. Several manufacturers produce toilets that wash the user with warm water and gently dry with warm air, eliminating the need for assistance to cleanse. It is advisable to check that products have Regulatory Approval (approved by the Water Regulations Advisory Scheme). The Alzheimer's Association (2006) web site provides brief details of skin care under the section of incontinence and toileting.

Special clothing

Impaired dexterity causes problems with fastenings and managing clothing. Altering the style of clothing will help, for example: elasticised waistbands and Velcro fastenings are easier than zips and buttons. The DLF's (2006f) fact sheet on *Clothing for Continence and Incontinence* provides guidelines and clothing suggestions for the management of catheters and urinals, including the use of drop-front, open-crotch and French knickers.

Incontinence garments and appliances

There are many incontinence garments and pads on the market, which are helpful in managing urinary incontinence. For infrequent light incontinence, when a small amount is voided, panty liners or sanitary pads may suffice. Alternatively, discreet and comfortable absorbent underpants can be used, washed and reused. Several have an effective absorbency of 100 ml or more and are suitable for light urinary incontinence. It is important to note that pads can cause skin rashes and the skin must be washed thoroughly.

Body-worn pads (Continence Foundation, 2005) and urine collecting devices are also available. Many different companies produce continence pads of varying absorbency, including ones specifically designed for men. The Medicines and Healthcare Products Regulatory Agency (described in Macaulay *et al.*, 2005) carried out an evaluation of 14 absorbent products for men with light urinary incontinence. Seventy-four men tested six 'leafs', six pouches, one pantegral, and one small pad. Leakage data was taken from 3,386 wet pads. Overall the leaf, pantegral, and small pad designs performed significantly better than the pouch. The evaluation report summarised the opinions of the 74 males tested. A 'leaf' design was found to be the best performing product.

NHS Direct (`http://www.nhsdirect.nhs.uk/`) provides details of the nearest continence service and advises on eligibility for free supplies.

Conclusion

It is important for care staff to look for reasons for incontinence, as environmental and behavioural factors may simply be the cause. It is often possible to facilitate continence by practical measures, including checking that mobility equipment is appropriate, ensuring that residents' bladders are never over-full and that they can locate and get to the toilet easily. Ensure that residents are able to manage their clothing.

Pelvic floor exercises are effective and can be incorporated into an activities programme. In a care home setting, it is essential to adopt a positive approach to toileting that treats people with dignity and respect. A tactful, sensitive approach is needed to preserve residents' self-esteem.

Key points

- Refer the resident for medical advice, as incontinence may be treatable.
- Environmental and behavioural factors can cause incontinence.
- Check that residents can manage the process of toileting.
- Talk to the residents about continence issues – several alternative solutions may be possible.
- Develop a toilet routine for individual residents.

Recreational activities

CHAPTER 18

The value of recreational activities

Leisure time enhances a sense of self and provides a balanced lifestyle. It is important to take opportunities to combine work, rest and play. When people retire and the running of a household is no longer the dominant consideration, there is often more time to enjoy hobbies and explore interests.

Today's generation of older people entering residential care have lived through a time where recreation has been an essential component of emotional, physical and cultural well-being. Thus people entering into residential care have generally had a lifestyle built predominantly around leisure, and the care regime needs to reflect this and provide opportunities to facilitate leisure pursuits.

Care standards

In the introduction to standards 12–15 of the *Care Homes for Older People: National Minimum Standards*, the Department of Health (2002a) highlights that:

- Social, cultural, recreational and occupational characteristics, which have taken a lifetime to emerge, do not suddenly disappear when individuals reach a later stage of life.
- A home's information pack should provide details of social life and its range of activities.
- Some people will want an active, well-organised social life, while others will want a level of privacy and independence from other residents.
- Many residents will need special support and assistance in engaging in the activities of daily life.

Valuing diversity

Everyone has a unique history, a portfolio of pastimes and personal interests. Individuals need a combination of recreational activities that recognises both social factors, as well as individual interests. Recreation is the component of life that enables individuals to exercise most choice. At work, there is frequently a need to suppress individuality for the collective good, but in leisure the choice is a purely personal one.

Facilitating recreational activities based upon a good assessment of need is a significant key to unlocking the inherent skills within individuals. A resident's profile, as outlined in Chapter 6 on assessment, enables a full assessment of need. By recognising older people's interests, people can be enabled to reach their full potential.

The key to any recreational activity, though, is the individuality of the process. People have different interests, and these should be respected. Individual choice may be influenced by people's cultural and religious backgrounds and opportunities need to be created to enable people to continue their previous interests. Furthermore, there is an opportunity to introduce people to new pursuits. These may be wide-ranging and diverse, from bingo to bonsai or dominoes to dancing!

Types of activity

The type of activity provided varies according to individual residents, the size of the group, the home and the availability of the care staff. Leisure activities can enhance our lives in many ways, for example:

- By expressing creativity (through art, craft, writing or dictating memoirs).
- By developing reflective activities through discussion and relaxation.
- By enhancing self-esteem when imparting skills and knowledge to others – for example, by instructing others or through reminiscence or music and literature discussions.
- By maintaining and improving physical abilities by active pastimes.

Often an activity has several benefits and individual needs can be met in a group activity. For example: the game of dominoes on a small group basis can be used to encourage individual social interaction, mental stimulation and communication. It can also encourage the use of hands, arm and trunk to improve manipulation skills, strength and balance. There are three basic types of activity:

- **Passive activities** – require slight participation from the residents but very little interaction. Examples are: aromatherapy, bird watching, listening to music, listening to talks from local people, massage, watching a concert or watching television.
- **Semi-active activities** – involve more participation. These include: crosswords, discussions, debates, quizzes, reminiscence, reality orientation or singing.
- **Active activities** – requiring more physical involvement from the residents. Examples are: art and craft, computer skills, cookery, dancing, gardening, local outings, movement to music, table games or yoga.

Some activities are individual and others are more group-focused. The list of activities is endless and will depend upon the resident's abilities and skills, as well as the care staff's skills and available resources, including budgets and facilities within the home.

How to start?

From an analysis of residents' profiles, some common interests can be identified and activities that people may wish to do can be established. Although with the normal processes of ageing the body will slow down, it is important to maximise the remaining functions and maintain a reasonable quality of life.

To enable residents to participate in leisure activities of their choice is an important goal, but it is also important to remember that residents may not want any active intervention. Some residents may be quite content with their current lifestyle. Not all residents wish to join in with group activities, but may need individual help to continue with their interests while in residential care. Some residents may join in for part of a session, while some people might choose not to join in at all. That is their choice and their right.

Samples of small group activities:
- Card games, e.g. rummy, whist, cribbage
- Table games, e.g. dominoes, bar skittles
- Art and craft
- Cookery, including 'no-cook' cookery
- Gardening, e.g. propagating plants, flower arrangements, potting plants
- Boules
- Reminiscence
- Meditation (cognitive quietening)
- Beauty and pampering sessions

Samples of larger group activities:

- Quizzes, e.g. family fortunes, proverb quizzes, music quizzes
- Movement to music, relaxation, Tai Chi, yoga
- Skittles
- Sing-a-longs

It may be impossible to cater for all needs, so a selection of activities within a recreation session is useful. To increase resources and stretch the budget, visitors can be asked for items, perhaps by putting up a strategically placed notice (Table 18.1).

The frailty of an individual should not prevent continuation of past interests. It is the process of leisure and the act of participation that is most significant, not the end result. There are many books that provide ideas for activities with residents. Start with a few activities and gradually build up a programme of activities. Use the 'KISS' principle – Keep It Simple and Safe!

Table 18.1 Items needed: wanted list.

Items needed

We are expanding our range of activities for residents.
If you have any of the following, please leave them at the office:

Art and craft materials
(poster or watercolour paints, small paintbrushes, wool, card, fabric, sequins, ribbons, watercolour paper)

Gardening equipment
(plant pots, compost, seeds, trowels)

Table games
(cards, scrabble, dominoes)

Quiz books

Any type of music CD

Small prizes
(soap, talc, ornaments etc.)

Thank you

Planning a session

There are no rules about the content of a session. However, a balanced programme that stimulates and encourages the maximum use of a resident's abilities should ideally provide:

- Social interaction (via group activity).
- Creative outlets (via practical-based activity).
- Mental stimulation and intellectual challenge (via table games and quizzes).
- Interaction with the local environment and community (through visits from local groups and through outings).
- Maximisation of a resident's level of physical function (through movement to music and other active pursuits).
- Continuation of pre-admission hobbies and interests.
- Maintenance of social and cultural links.

Adaptation of activities

Many leisure activities can be undertaken by using a different technique, such as sitting rather than standing to play bowls and changing hand preference. The possibilities are limitless and all staff can be encouraged to come up with suggested solutions to overcome problems.

- **Writing**

If hand function is impaired, for example due to a stroke or rheumatoid arthritis, writing can cause problems. Attachments can be provided on pens and writing implements to enlarge the gripping surface. Non-slip matting can be placed beneath a thin card or a clipboard can be used to stop paper slipping. A clipboard could be kept in the office so that if any signatures are required.

- **Craft activities**

Often a different technique can be used – for example, when painting, abstract images can be created. Small paintings are quick to do and can be turned into beautiful greeting cards. If the resident has difficulty holding paper, anchor the paper to the surface or use a clipboard. Larger brushes can be used or the handles can be padded if the ability to grip is limited. Small clamps can be used to fasten items to the table.

■ **Card games**

Card games can be difficult to join in when there is a problem holding cards. It is difficult to hold a hand and play when you only have the use of one hand. A DIY card holder can be made using an oblong tin and a few large elastic bands or a clean scrubbing brush turned upside down, perhaps stabilised on a piece of non-slip material. Alternatively, there are some excellent cardholders available.

■ **Practical activities**

These do not need to be completed in one session and some can be broken down into simple stages – a mini 'production line' can be created.

Implications for the home

The starting point for developing a positive approach to recreation is for the management to create an environment that encourages active participation. Care is not just focusing on meeting people's personal care needs. A total quality culture needs to be adopted by all staff and if group activities are being carried out, everyone has a part to play. Although one member of staff takes the session, the others need to be supportive – perhaps by helping to set up the session, being on toileting duty or taking an individual activity with another resident.

Activities need to be flexible and meet the resident's needs at that moment in time. Recreation is not purely a tool of occupation or diversion, but recognised by all concerned as being integral to providing good quality care that is holistic in approach.

If the environment meets people's higher social expectations, apart from the positive impact on individual residents, a home will look more attractive to potential future residents. This can be included in marketing materials showing residents engaged in leisure pursuits and enjoying themselves.

Conclusion

Leisure is a vital part of daily life, whether in a passive, semi-active or active way. Homes should view the provision of recreational activities as an essential part of maintaining and caring for residents' needs. Where relevant, activities should be linked to the resident's individual care plan. A home, through a structured approach to recreation, will improve the quality of life of its residents.

Key points

- Activities are not just provided to play a diversion or a time-filling role.
- Recreation can be a therapeutic experience.
- Residents should have a choice of activities and diversity valued.
- Some coaxing may be required, but residents have the right to not participate.
- Individual and group activities should be available.
- Build up sessions slowly to create a varied weekly programme.

CHAPTER 19

Gardening: a pleasurable and beneficial activity

With ageing or impairment of function, many heavy domestic tasks, including strenuous gardening jobs, can become a burden or impossible to achieve. For many people who enter a care home, there is a sense of relief, as garden maintenance is no longer their responsibility. There can, however, be a corresponding sense of loss at no longer having the pleasure of tending plants and seeing growth and new life emerge. This need not be the case.

With thought and attention paid to creative ways of undertaking garden activities, it is possible to enable residents in care homes to continue gardening. Also, people who did not have a garden or time to develop an interest before entering into a care environment can be helped to enjoy this pursuit.

The benefits of gardening to maintain and improve physical fitness and mental health are well known (Table 19.1). Foster and Powell (1992) state: 'Gardening is a healthful way to reduce frustration, anxiety and stress and increase receptiveness to the approach of other people'. Gardening can be used to help to channel aggressive feelings into productive behaviours.

Table 19.1 Benefits of gardening (Better Health Channel, 2005).

- An enjoyable form of exercise.
- Increases levels of physical activity and maintains mobility and flexibility.
- Encourages use of all motor skills (walking, reaching and bending) through activities such as planting seeds and taking cuttings.
- Improves endurance and strength.
- Helps prevent diseases like osteoporosis.
- Reduces stress levels and promotes relaxation.
- Provides stimulation and interest in nature and the outdoors.
- Improves well-being as a result of social interaction.

All levels of ability

Although gardening activities can maintain and improve physical abilities, a garden can purely be a place to sit in, to socialise in, or simply to look out on. Gardening can be enjoyed by people with no former knowledge of horticulture, and provide a new interest or hobby at many levels of ability. Residents can take part in the planning stages if areas are redesigned or a bed is replanted, or participate in a more active, physical manner.

People who have tended plants have a wealth of experience and knowledge to share, from how to grow cuttings successfully to prevention of disease and pest control. A resident may wish to take care of a single plant, perhaps in their private room, or want to help tend a section of the communal garden.

Some homes have patio doors leading from a bedroom area, and the areas around are landscaped to a resident's preference or planters placed within reach of the resident. Strategically placed trowels can be left in raised beds to encourage residents to 'potter' in the garden.

Health and safety aspects

Although gardening is pleasurable experience, it can cause many problems for residents, and care is needed. Causes of falling incidents include uneven paving or changes in level. A risk assessment should include mobility and

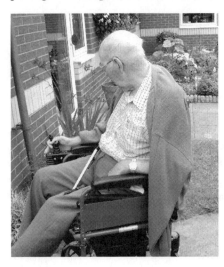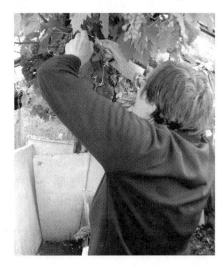

Gardening: a passive or active experience (© Julie Swann 2007 (left) and NRC 2006 (right)).

safety within the outside environment, particularly if there are any potential hazards, such as steps within the grounds or access to a road.

Often, when engrossed in an activity, poor posture and bad habits can occur and lead to strains. Ergonomic or adapted tools make tasks easier and safer. It is a good idea to do some gentle stretching exercises before gardening, as with any physical activity. Encourage residents to move around and alternate larger movements with smaller movements. It is important to encourage regular rests and not to sit slouched, nor rest on one leg or one arm for long periods when gardening. Residents should be encouraged to drink plenty of decaffeinated fluids to prevent dehydration, and take breaks in the shade.

Skin sensitivity

Some medication, including major tranquillisers, increases skin sensitivity; it is important for care staff to know if residents need to take extra care of their skin to avoid burning in summer months. Loose, long-sleeved tops, wide-brimmed hats and high factor sunscreen should be used as protection from the hot summer rays.

Providing shade

Trees and shrubs can provide natural shade. Many care homes have umbrellas or chairs sited beneath the shade provided by a wall. Wooden pergolas can be attached to a wall and provide a roof for sitting under and keeping the house cool in summer by shading windows from the sun. Climbers scrambling over will soften the effect and provide additional shade and privacy (Newstead, 2004). During summer months gazebos provide shade, while in the darker winter months they can be removed and stowed away. Gazebos can be purchased from many garden centres and high street stores. A wall-hung pull-down canopy (folding awning) provides a transitional space between inside and outside. Many modern canopies are architectural features that add sculptural, yet practical features to garden settings.

Planning the right time

Some residents prefer hotter temperatures, like the warmth that a greenhouse environment provides to arthritic hands, whilst others may prefer the cool of the shade. Some residents may be more mobile at certain times of the day; for example: residents with Parkinson's disease may have 'on–off' moments. The Arthritis Foundation (2006) advises people to:

> plan to garden during the times of day when you feel best; for example, wait until afternoon if you have morning stiffness. That way you'll be able to work more easily and will enjoy it more than if you're stiff or sore.

Problem areas

Practical care of plants requires some motor control and coordination. Some residents may have lost some range of movement and strength, which can pose problems with gardening. However, easier-to-manage tools (e.g. with long handles) and products are available in several supermarkets, DIY stores and high street shops. Gipp (2005) explains that it makes a great deal of sense for everyone to consider tools, methods and techniques that help reduce stress, strain, effort – and possibly injury, whatever their age.

Ergonomically designed lightweight tools reduce stress on joints and muscles. Many garden tools (Yeoman and Spear & Jackson) are available from garden centres or specialist companies, such as Darlac (http://www.darlac.com/) and Gardena (http://www.gardena.co.uk/). Several products on the market are aimed at middle-aged gardening enthusiasts, with their spending power and leisure time. These products are also useful for residents with physical problems. The charity Disability Norfolk will provide information and advice on DIY solutions and has a useful, inspirational article on *Gardening with Disabilities* (http://www.bbc.co.uk/norfolk/your/access/disability/index.shtml).

DIY solutions

Many problem areas can be minimised by good design and through the provision of adapted tools or DIY solutions (Table 19.2). Tools can be altered with very little cost:

Table 19.2 Solutions to gardening problems.

Problem	Solution
Bending to ground level and back problems.	Long-handled 'dibber' and long-handled reacher Quick-release multi-change long-handled tools, including snap-on, twist-on and clip-on tool heads Raised beds Long-handled planters or use short sections of drainpipe Spades with 'T' handles to avoid twisting and causing back pain Double-handled grips attached to tools to allow both hands to be used, thus reducing pressure on the back Pacing tasks and allowing for rest, or doing less strenuous activities Working at 'trunk' level or from a seated position Avoiding lifting, holding or carrying heavy items Using an old walking stick as a 'dibber'
Limited standing ability	Use of a patio chair or gardening stool to sit to do tasks Raised beds with sufficient width to sit on top edge 'Table top' gardening
Wheelchair users	Long-handled tools and raised beds
Generalised weakness	Lightweight tools Tools with greater leverage Using light, easily worked soil Container gardening, indoors and outdoors
Difficulty reaching up	Long-handled pruners or secateurs made from lightweight aluminium
Left-handed user	Left-handed tools
Impaired grip	Easy-grip appliances Ratchet-type pruners Padded handles on hand tools Using gloves with 'gripper dots' Universal cuff that attaches to the arm or forearm so that a lightweight tool can be attached
One-handed use	Cut-and-hold tools, e.g. flower gatherer or pruner Placing a wheelbarrow beneath pruning area Toolbar strapped around the waist
Loss of dexterity	Using 'seed strips', pellets, 'click seeders' or a flour shaker to distribute seeds
Poor vision	Brightly coloured tools Larger or pellet seeds Using tactile or scented plants
Cognitive problems and mild confusional states	Simple garden layout with focal points Using way-finding signage Using plants that will trigger positive memories Awareness of the dangers from gardening equipment, including trip hazards from hosepipes and tools Avoiding 'dangerous' plants that cause problems if ingested or brushed against

- Wheelchair users and seated gardeners can use a short piece of guttering or a drainpipe to help when planting clumps of plants, bulbs or to 'plug' seedlings and plants.
- Lightweight tubing such as narrow plastic pipes can be used to bed seeds.
- A short broom handle can help with placement and a 'soil-pusher' can be made from a short broom handle and a small rectangle of wood.
- Fishing net can be used in conjunction with a long-handled tool to extract plants and items from ground level (if a long-handled wooden tool is too heavy, use aluminium or plastic tubing).

Activities linked to gardening

Gardening need not be confined to the outdoor growing season or environment, as indoor houseplants also need attention. Activities related to gardening can be incorporated into an activities programme. Woodwork projects could include the assembly of birdhouses, window boxes and raised planters. Late autumn and winter months can be used to plan for the next season and to refurbish or preserve containers.

Cuttings can be taken, seeds propagated and plants re-potted outside of the outdoor growing season. The material grown in a garden is useful for flower arranging in fresh and dried forms; dried materials can be used in many art and craft activities.

Visits outside of the care environment could include garden centres, National Trust property and stately home gardens. A list of gardens to visit in the UK is provided by Great British Gardens (http://www.greatbritishgardens.co.uk/index.htm). This web site provides details of disabled access, cafés and facilities.

Conclusion

With inclusive garden design and suitable tools, residents with limited mobility or those who have problems with manual dexterity and strength can take part in gardening activities. There is a wide range of equipment that can be obtained to help make gardening a pleasurable task and with ingenuity, DIY solutions can be found to many problem areas. Gardening is an activity that stimulates all of the senses and is adaptable to individual needs either by using different tools or techniques.

Key points

- Gardening is a pleasurable and therapeutic activity for many.
- It can be carried out indoors or outdoors.
- Many adapted tools are available to facilitate this activity.
- Raised beds are useful for all age ranges and disabilities.
- Gardening can be an active or sedentary activity.

CHAPTER 20

Cognitive quietening: turning down the mind's clock

Relaxation is important to help minds and bodies de-stress after strenuous or prolonged activity and to help unwind before they go to sleep. Some people use several activities or techniques to help with relaxation, ranging from active exercise and purposeful activity to sedentary, or indeed often meaningless, activity. Everyone relaxes in a different way.

When planning an activities programme, it is important to include some relaxing pastimes for residents. Table 20.1 indicates some of the activities commonly used to 'chill out'. Each activity has its own benefits, yet the general theme is one of relaxation and cognitive quietening. Several activities that are used to relax cost very little, except for staff time.

Table 20.1 Some activities used for relaxation.

Listening to relaxing music	Changing into comfortable clothes
Watching television, video or DVD	Having a pampering session
Reading	Massage
Drinking or eating	Beauty/skin treatments
Talking to someone, particularly venting your feelings	Reflexology
Sleeping (40 winks)	Aromatherapy
Playing cards	Taking a bath
Reflection	Hobbies
Practising breathing slowly, breathing exercises and deep breathing	Progressive muscular relaxation techniques
Meditation/imagery	Gardening
Writing a diary or creative writing	Dancing or moving to music
Daydreaming	Singing
Stroking pets	Gentle exercise or strolling
'Watching the world go by'	Yoga, Tai Chi or pilates

As well as being an enjoyable activity, relaxation techniques can also be used to help residents (and staff) cope with stress.

Acute stress response

Walter Cannon first described the fight or flight response, also called the 'acute stress response', in 1929. The theory states that animals react to threats with a general discharge of the sympathetic nervous system. An animal therefore has two options when faced with danger: it can either face the threat (fight) or it can avoid the threat (flight). A fight or flight response is therefore the body's automatic response to a perception of danger. The response was later recognised as the first stage of a general adaptation syndrome that regulates stress responses among vertebrates and other organisms.

Types of relaxation technique

Relaxation techniques are broadly grouped into those acting on the physical body and those that act on the mind. Smith (2005) describes physical relaxation as yoga stretches, progressive muscular relaxation (PMR) and breathing exercises, with mental activities being autogenic suggestion, meditation, imagery and relaxing self-talk.

Relaxation techniques like meditation, yoga and Tai Chi have been used for centuries. This chapter concentrates on two main relaxation activities that care staff can carry out on a group or an individual basis with residents – yoga and relaxation. It is essential to check with the general practitioner, to ascertain whether any particular movements are contraindicated for individual residents.

■ **Yoga stretches**
Yoga has three main components: body posture, breathing and meditation. Many yoga postures consist of stretches that can be carried out while lying on a bed or when sitting in a chair. Folliard (2006) describes many chair-based postures with visual images. Several yoga postures can be adapted to non-ambulant (seated) people. Many yoga stretches can be carried out while lying on a bed or when sitting in a chair. Kent (1985) provides visual images of yoga postures, showing how these can be modified for wheelchair users and people with physical problems. Care must be taken when forward postures are car-

ried out, as feet should be on the floor or on a raised surface, not on footrests – otherwise, the wheelchair may tip forwards.

■ **Progressive muscle relaxation (PMR)**

In the 1930s, Edmund Jacobson, a physiologist and psychologist, pioneered PMR. He based this upon his premise that mental calmness is a natural result of physical relaxation (Jacobson, 1938). Today, PMR is used after classes like yoga, Tai Chi or pilates. PMR is an effective method of pain relief and can reduce anxiety and to help with insomnia. If techniques are successful, they may help residents to reduce the amount of sedation and other medication they need. PMR consists of tensing and relaxing each muscle group, with a final couple of minutes of focusing on visual imagery or relaxing to gentle music.

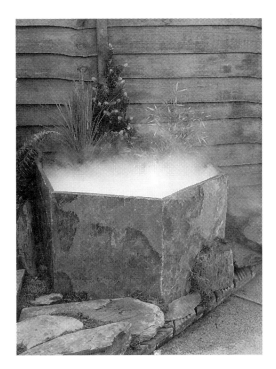

Meditation: focusing on objects (© NRC 2006).

Where to do relaxation

Ideally, relaxation should be carried out in a warm, quiet room that is free from distractions. Participants either lie in a 'corpse' posture (on the back with hands held loosely at the side and legs outstretched) or sit comfortably in a chair. Emphasis is placed on slow, long breathing. At the end of a session, participants are taken through some gentle stretches to 'wake up' again.

Relaxation activities require very little cost and relaxation can be carried out on an individual or group basis; for example:

- A short session focusing on breathing, aimed at residents with breathing problems or limited lung capacity.
- Five to 15 minutes relaxation at the end of an activities session or before bedtime.
- A PMR session lasting up to 60 minutes, depending on the resident group.

There are many books, such as Fallon-Goodhew (2002), and resources on the Internet that provide a longer relaxation 'script', for example that provided by the University of Florida at http://www.relaxation.com/relaxation-exercises.htm. Quarta (2001) describes Tai Chi, which can be carried out in a chair.

Referring to the last step in Table 20.2: visualisation may stimulate, not quieten, an active mind – so encourage the participants to think of being inside a warm comfortable bed or to sink into the folds of a deep, dark, velvet curtain.

Table 20.2 A basic relaxation exercise to try.

- Choose a quiet place where you won't be interrupted.
- Before you start, do a few gentle stretching exercises to relieve muscular tension.
- Make yourself comfortable, either sitting or lying down.
- Start to breathe slowly and deeply, in a calm and effortless way.
- Gently tense, and then relax each part of the body, starting with the feet and working up to the face and head.
- When focusing on each area, think of warmth, heaviness and relaxation.
- Push any distracting thoughts to the back of the mind; imagine them floating away.
- Don't try to relax, simply let go of the tension in the muscles and allow them to become relaxed.
- Let the mind go empty (some find it helpful to visualise a calm, beautiful place such as a garden or meadow).
- Stay like this for about 20 minutes, then take some deep breaths and open the eyes, but stay sitting or lying for a few moments before getting up (Tighe, 2006).

Other relaxation techniques

There are many other types of relaxation activity that can be adapted to be used within a care setting, including mini relaxation techniques, breathing exercises, autogenic suggestion, meditation, imagery and mental rehearsal.

■ Mini relaxation techniques

These can be useful if people are under stress of any type, particularly if a person suffers from panic attacks. Examples are provided in Table 20.3. Care staff may find these useful when they are in stressful situations, including preparing for a job interview, doing a presentation or when dealing with a difficult situation. Webster (1996) writes that mini relaxation exercises are focused breathing techniques, which help reduce anxiety and tension immediately.

■ Breathing exercises

The chest carries out shallow chest breathing and the abdomen carries out deep breathing. Deep breathing is a simple yet effective method of relaxing.

Breathing should be calm and regular and intakes of breath can be given colour and qualities – for example, a relaxing intake of 'blue' air or an intake of energising 'red' air. Breathing exercises can improve respiratory function and relieve stress, tension and anxiety, but care should be taken to avoid hyperventilation and dizziness.

■ Autogenic suggestion

A cue, such as a word or mental image associated with calmness, is used to trigger feelings of muscle relaxation – for example: warmth, lakes, mountains, floating on air.

Table 20.3 Mini relaxation techniques.

- Squeeze the eyes tight and clench teeth, shoulders, buttocks, legs and toes.
- Hold the body tight for a count of three, then let go completely.
- Repeat twice, then breath easily.

(Adapted from Fallon-Goodhew, 2002)

- Focus on a place, person or word that evokes a pleasurable feeling or a peaceful scene and breathe in deeply and slowly, then breathe out. Take another deep breath and let it out; feel yourself release the tensions in your mind and in your body.

■ Meditation

Meditation is found in several of the major religions, including Christianity, Buddhism, Hinduism and Islam. It ranges from control of breathing to focusing on objects (such as an ornament or flower), a word or a phrase that is associated with pleasure or calmness (similar to autogenic suggestion). A syllable or word is repeated silently or in a low, gentle tone recited in time with breathing (mantra). Repetition is used to reduce logical, externally oriented thoughts by focusing solely on this one stimulus. Thoughts, feelings and other images are encouraged to drift away while relaxation is carried out for 5–20 minutes and the mind focuses on a feeling of calmness. Benson (1975) carried out a series of experiments in 1968 using meditation and found these techniques reduced stress and controlled the fight or flight response. He found that meditation slowed heartbeat and breathing, reduced oxygen consumption and aided relaxation.

■ Imagery, guided imagery and relaxing self-talk

Imagery can involve all the senses (hearing, sight, smell, taste and touch). For example, imagine a woodland scene, a beach, a waterfall or birds flying. Relaxation tapes are available in many music outlets with gentle music or tranquil, natural sounds, such as water or bird sounds, which help to promote feelings of relaxation. Guided imagery can focuses on past pleasant experiences or new situations.

■ Mental rehearsal

Mental rehearsal involves imagining a situation or scenario then thinking of an ideal outcome. It can be used to reduce anxiety about a forthcoming situation or important event. The idea is to imagine each step of the anxiety-provoking event and successfully manage to complete it. Barnes's (2004) chapter on enhancing techniques describes mental rehearsals, including techniques to diffuse excessive energy and reduce anxiety.

Conclusion

Relaxation is an important aspect of life and a useful part of a recreational programme within a care setting. Most relaxation techniques can be carried out at any time and in any place, and have been used for decades in the treatment of anxiety and panic attacks. Relaxation techniques have obvious benefits for residents who are easily stressed or mildly agitated residents to help produce calmness.

PMR is a helpful technique for staff and residents to use. PMR can be combined with deep breathing and visualisation of a safe comfortable place to relax into. Relaxation is an important aspect of modern day life and is an important part of a recreational programme within a care setting.

Key points

■ The ability to relax can vary from day to day.

■ Try a range of techniques to find out which one works best on individual people.

■ Choose a quiet comfortable place.

■ Residents may prefer a 5–10 minute individual session than a group activity.

CHAPTER 21

Pampering and basic skin care

Beauty products and treatments are no longer just for the wealthy; today, skin care is considered to be an essential part of daily life. Throughout the world many people use products to keep their skin in good condition. High street chemists, supermarkets, department stores, mail order outlets and the 'bargain' shops stock extensive ranges of products for skin care. Many are designed to suit various skin types for all ages and both sexes; with increasing ranges specifically aimed at men. Residents often spend considerable time indoors and central heating tends to dry out older, thin and fragile skin.

Facial, hand and foot care is already provided to residents as part of personal grooming, but it is possible to develop this personal care task into a pampering session. Some care homes are already doing this as part of individual or small group activities. No formal training is needed for skin care routines, as they are basic common sense. A 'pampering afternoon' can be made to be part of an activities programme, where residents are encouraged to apply some products themselves.

Types of pampering session

Although massage is a skilled technique, in its simplest form, massage of the face, hand or foot is something anyone can do. Basic skin care can be transformed into a beauty treatment with very little extra effort:

- Application of facial moisturiser – becomes a facial massage.
- Application of cleanser, toner and moisturiser – becomes a deep cleansing facial.
- Application of foot cream – becomes a foot massage.
- General hand care – becomes a hand massage.
- Washing hair – becomes a deep conditioning treatment and scalp massage.
- Getting ready to go out – becomes a subtle application of cosmetics.

In this way, general care of individuals can be transformed into a pleasurable pampering session, with the obvious pleasurable benefits for residents.

Cost to the home

Most residents will already have basic skin care products, with towels and other items in supply within the home. Several homes have underused hairdressing salons or rooms that would be ideal for an individual or small group beauty session. The real economic cost of individual sessions is the additional staff time spent with residents. This can be beneficial in its own right, as relationships can develop during the activity and care is provided in a way that is more participative and relaxed. However, where staff time is at a premium it is possible to contact local colleges who may run NVQ courses in beauty therapy. This provides a five-fold benefit:

- Residents: gain opportunities to take part in pampering sessions and interact with other people who are outside of their environment.
- The college: gains work placements for their students.
- The students: gain models, providing hands-on experience of caring for the skin.
- The care home: benefits from additional people to do the pampering sessions, although some supervision will be needed.
- Care staff: can sit in on sessions and learn new techniques and ideas.

Factors to consider during sessions

Although no formal training is required, there are a few basic factors to consider in setting up a pampering session. These include:

- Ensure the residents are comfortable and relaxed.
- Use a warm room.
- Have everything at hand ready to use.
- Keep your nails short if you are applying products.
- Avoid jewellery and keep long hair tied back.
- Wear loose clothing.
- Ensure that any products used are suitable for the resident's skin.
- Safely store aromatherapy or beauty products that can cause an adverse reaction if ingested, or may irritate delicate skin.
- Chat to the resident; but do not talk unnecessarily if you are doing an individual session, as this can hinder relaxation.
- Provide some background music when taking a group session.

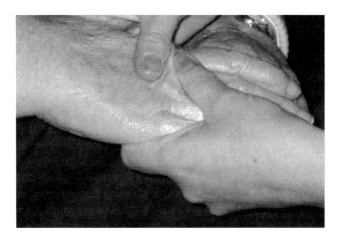

Applying cream: gentle hand massage (© NRC 2006).

When considering products to apply, care is needed with sensitive skin as some ingredients, e.g. essential oils, may irritate the skin. Either use products designed for sensitive skins or do a 'patch test' inside the wrist and leave this for 12 hours. Care must be taken if there is any skin disease, open cuts or abrasions, bruising, allergic reactions or highly vascular skin (Cressy, 2003). If an adverse reaction occurs, cleanse immediately with almond oil then wash the area. Dry or mature skin will benefit from a rich cream that blends in easily and glides on, i.e. does not drag the skin. However, skin care is not just about re-moisturising, as some residents (such as people with Parkinson's disease) may have an increase of secretions, leading to excessively oily skin.

The benefits of massage

There are many physical, physiological and psychological benefits in a basic massage. If the correct products are applied, the skin will become nourished and the skin texture will improve. The underlying muscles will become toned and cellular regeneration is encouraged. Massage is also an excellent method of relaxation.

Many residents have limited physical contract from others, often only during personal care and help with mobility. Holding, touching and comforting can be given in a socially acceptable and appropriate manner through 'hands-on' beauty care. Maxwell-Hudson (1999) explains that touch and massage are forms of non-verbal communication that help nurses to establish empathy and understanding with their patients. This concept applies across the care sector. Karrie Osborn (2004) notes:

> It took time, but eventually my grandmother began looking forward to seeing the massage volunteer who brought oils and strong hands to nurse her feet and ankles. She told me how good the massage made her feel, and while I knew that the therapy certainly helped her arthritic body, I also knew that her greatest comfort came in simply being touched by another human being.

Gender and cultural issues

As with all activities, it is important to recognise that there may be issues related to gender and/or cultural issues. These should be carefully considered especially when planning any hands on activity.

Techniques of massage

Massage techniques are found in many books on beauty therapy, including NVQ textbooks. One of the massage techniques, effleurage, is a soothing, stroking, surface movement and can be safely given by care staff as it is similar to application of creams and emollients. Petrissage (deep pressure movement), tapotement (tapping and digital hacking) and vibrations (fine trembling movements) should be left to a qualified masseur. Toselli (2005) provides a pictorial step-by-step guide to massage, face, foot and hand care. Several mediums can be used for massage (Cressy, 2003), including:

- Oils (providing they are light, non-sticky and easily absorbed); for example olive oil and almond oils.
- Essential aromatherapy oils, extracted from plants, can be mixed with suitable carrier oils that are easily absorbed and odourless, for example grape seed, avocado, almond and wheat germ. Suitable essential oils include camomile, cypress, ylang-ylang, sandalwood, patchouli, rose, neroli and lavender.
- Massage creams contain specific ingredients to suit all skin types and are ready mixed for application.

Key points to remember when giving a massage

Crowther (1996) provides some key points for the person giving the massage:

- Be aware of posture to avoid straining.
- Lengthen the spine and neck with every movement.
- Do not hunch the shoulders.
- Keep the back flat when bending forwards.
- Stop immediately if any massage step is uncomfortable or causes pain.

Some massages to try with residents:

- **Facial massage**

Facial massages are easier to carry out if the resident is seated and you are at the back of their chair. The massage medium should help fingers and hands to glide over the skin. First warm your hands, then warm the massage medium in your hands. Apply massage medium in rhythmical movements for up to 20 minutes, taking care to avoid overstretching or over stimulation of tissue. Reapply massage medium if your hands feel as though they are dragging.

- **Hand massage**

This can be carried out after a hand soak in warm soapy water or a bath. The carer should sit alongside the resident, and a table top used to provide additional support for the hand or the hand rested upon a towel placed on the resident's knee.

- **Foot massage**

Foot massage may be preceded by a bath or a foot soak in a spa bath. The resident's foot should be elevated either by using a footstool or by carrying out the massage with the person lying on the bed.

Aromatherapy

The benefits of fragrance to re-energise and stimulate or to relax and calm are well known. Aromatherapy is the systematic use of essential oils in holistic treatments to improve physical and emotional well-being, and aromatherapy products can be used for massage. Several ready mixed aromatherapy products are available in the high street. These are basically a mixture of carrier oil and an essential oil. All-purpose carrier oils include apricot kernel oil and sunflower oil. There are special carrier oils that improve penetration of products into skin, such as avocado oil, wheat germ oil and jojoba (Maxwell-Hudson, 1999). Useful essential oils are:

- Facial care: sandalwood, rose, bergamot and chamomile
- Foot care: peppermint, teatree oil
- Hand care: geranium

Aromatherapy, like massage, is a highly skilled art. Qualified aromatherapists belonging to a professional association can be located at http://www.aromatherapy-regulation.org.uk/. All aromatherapists should be insured to practice and abide by a code of conduct and ethics supported by disciplinary procedures.

Care staff are therefore advised to use ready prepared products rather than make their own mixes, as the ratio of essential oil to carrier oil is important. For example: for normal skin, ten drops of essential oil to 20 ml of carrier oil are used; for sensitive skin, five drops of essential oil to 20 ml of carrier oil are used; for very sensitive skin, one drop of essential oil to 20 ml of carrier oil is recommended (Maxwell-Hudson, 1999).

Residents who are confused may mistake essential oils for medicine, so only have small quantities of pre-mixed oil in places accessible by residents.

Myatt (2005) outlines the other uses of aromatherapy products, including inhalation and pillow oils, and provides a starter list of oils and their uses.

Conclusion

Pampering is an essential part of modern-day life and is used to refresh or relax. There are many skin care products easily available in local outlets or by mail order. Residents may already have personal preferences, with an array of products in their personal belongings. By spending a little more time in the application of skin care products, care staff can turn basic skin care into a pampering session that will have positive effects for residents, who will be encouraged to feel good about their physical appearance.

Key points

- Pampering improves general well-being.
- Sessions can be carried out on a group or individual basis.
- Facial, hand and foot massages are relaxing.
- Products are readily available in many local outlets.
- The benefits of aromatherapy to relax or to re-energise are well known.

PART 9

Keeping mobile

PART 2

Keeping mobile

CHAPTER 22

Helping individuals keep mobile

Movement is a complex process, and many people encounter difficulties moving within and outside their home. Some problems associated with ageing can cause impairment of mobility, but difficulties can be minimised. The emphasis of intervention is on the provision of the right amount of assistance to maintain, and in many cases improve, a person's level of mobility.

Moving effectively

Execution of movement patterns is a highly refined skill. To move effectively requires precise input from several sensory neurological pathways in the body, such as:

- Proprioception (to help register where limbs are in relation to other bodily parts)
- Vestibular (inner ear mechanisms and their connections within the brain stem assist balance)
- Visual and auditory pathways (helps to negotiate the surrounding environment)
- Tactile information (assists the sensory detection of walking surfaces, arm rests, walking aids and handrails)

Information collected via sensory pathways is processed within the brain. Some aspects of movement are dealt with subconsciously, as with breathing, or automatically, such as digestion and heart rate. Basic reflex actions, for example knee jerks, are controlled at the spinal cord level. For moving around, however, the action is a conscious process requiring individuals to use a combination of complex cognitive and physical abilities in a coordinated fashion. With ageing or the onset of disabling conditions these processes may become impaired or simply underused.

Mobility problems

Mobility is often construed as an ability to walk. However, mobility has a much wider connotation. It is used to describe any movement pattern and range of movement that a joint is capable of achieving. The ability to be mobile is often taken for granted even when longstanding abnormal movement and gait patterns are present. Some residents have multiple problems that are superimposed on each other: for example, they may suffer from a stroke superimposed on heart and orthopaedic conditions. Loss of agility, due to gradual wear and tear caused by ageing, can further restrict the level of mobility. Maintaining mobility requires a certain level of physical and cognitive ability and motivation is a major factor. Mobility difficulties may occur as a result of the following problems:

■ **Muscular problems**
Weakness can be caused by generalised ill-heath, specific muscle damage or damage to the nerves supplying a muscle. An increase in muscle tone (spasticity) will prevent full range of movement. This may occur if, for example, the individual has suffered a severe stroke or has multiple sclerosis.

■ **Joint problems**
Gradual wear and tear of the cartilage (as in osteoarthritis), ligament problems (for example, 'frozen' shoulder) or injury to a joint (such as, a fracture) can cause orthopaedic problems. The joint can become inflamed, as is the case in rheumatoid arthritis or gout. Joints can become painful or swollen, further restricting movement.

■ **Impairment of nerve supply**
If a motor nerve is impaired as a result of injury (for example, peripheral nerve injury or spinal injury) muscles will not function properly. In multiple sclerosis, damage to the myelin sheath that surrounds the nerve reduces the conductivity of nerve impulses, causing problems with coordination and balance.

■ **Fatigue, drowsiness and lethargy**
Several medical conditions, including viral infections, cause fatigue, lethargy and a general reduction in mobility. Some medication can cause unsteadiness and difficulty initiating movement. Tranquillisers promote drowsiness and muscle weakness and blunt the postural reflexes (Vassallo *et al.*, 2004). Any side effects should be reported to a doctor.

■ **Cognitive problems**
A reduction in cognitive abilities causes difficulties in understanding instructions and a reduction in awareness of personal safety.

■ Sensory problems

Sensory problems are not only confined to visual or hearing loss. Some people have severe numbness in their feet and are unable to feel the floor or know where their feet are when walking.

Awareness

It is important to be aware of the origin of movement problems, as this can influence the type of intervention required to assist an individual. Although problems can be short term, ligaments and muscle tendons can tighten unless exercised. Compensatory patterns of movement, which may in the long term create problems, are soon learned. Assistance provided by staff should focus on general mobility and encouraging residents to keep all of their limbs working by stretching and maintaining flexibility. In addition to working on a specific joint or area of the body, exercise has several supplementary benefits. Regular physical activity decreases the risk of coronary heart disease, stroke and diabetes, and the associated risk factors such as hypertension and obesity (Department of Health, 2007).

Staff development

Managers of care homes need to have an awareness of movement problems and should encourage care staff to develop an appreciation of the difficulties that residents may experience. This is encapsulated in training, as to complete the NVQ level 2 unit in care titled 'Enabling individuals to keep mobile' candidates must show sufficient levels of competence in the following elements:

a. Support individuals to keep mobile.
b. Observe any changes in the individual's mobility and provide feedback to the appropriate people.

Providing support

Supporting people to keep mobile is more than assisting a person to stand and walk; it is important to keep arms and trunk muscles mobile, as well as the legs. Proactive support involves providing physical assistance, utilising assistive devices, providing encouragement and ensuring that the environment facilitates safe mobilisation. These four approaches are described below.

Providing physical assistance

Physical assistance should be provided when needed, with residents encouraged to do as much as possible for themselves. If a chair is too low, rising will become difficult. If a chair is too high the circulation to the legs can be compromised. Seat heights of chairs or beds should allow the thighs to be parallel to the floor, and be firm yet comfortable.

Before attempting to help a person to stand, ensure that footwear is suitable, supportive and fastened. Feet can swell due to circulatory problems, causing footwear to cut into the flesh; larger sizes or footwear with elasticised fastenings can be used. The appliance department of the local hospital can raise shoes, trainers and slippers, for example if there is limb length discrepancy or the Achilles tendon at the heel shortens. Tendon shortening is common in people with lower limb spasticity (e.g. post-stroke, head injury or suffering from multiple sclerosis).

It is important to assess how much a resident can self-mobilise before offering direct physical support. The 'get-up and go test' (Mathias *et al.*, 1986) requires patients to stand up from a chair, walk a short distance, turn around, return, and sit down again.

Often techniques just need to be reinforced. Encourage the resident to move forwards to the firm front edge of the seat. Residents should not be pulled up into a standing position or given a hand to hold. Both their hands should be placed on the arms of the chair in preparation for standing, even if physical assistance to stand is provided. Check that both feet are flat on the ground. As the knees move forward in the action of standing do not 'block' the knee, as this hinders the ability to stand.

Assistive devices

Assistive devices may be needed to maximise independence and assist a resident to move into a standing position (Table 22.1). These items can be used in a care home or if residents return to the community.

Table 22.1 Some solutions to transferring problems.

Turning in bed	Glide sheets Monkey pole Bed handrails
Getting from lying to sitting position	Bed rope ladder Pillow/mattress lifter Monkey pole Bed handrails
Rising into standing	Check bed/chair height Ensure seat unit/mattress is firm enough to push up from Floor to ceiling poles sited by bed Chair risers Riser units on chairs Electric riser chairs

Providing encouragement

Care staff can encourage mobility and reinforce good patterns of movement when carrying out basic personal care activities, as well as when walking with residents. Residents should be encouraged to be as self-managing as possible. Prolonged sitting should be avoided as this can cause pressure areas; muscles can atrophy (waste away) and tendons can tighten, causing loss of range of movement and muscle power.

When standing and sitting, arm and trunk muscles bring the body into position. When walking leg, trunk and arm movements are used to achieve a normal gait pattern.

Many homes have visiting therapists and care staff can carry out activities between therapy sessions. It is important to carry over movements into an activity, e.g. reaching and bending movements can be incorporated into a recreational activity. Gentle exercise and encouraging residents to participate in activities within the care home is the role of an activities coordinator, but all care staff can encourage and facilitate residents outside of structured sessions.

Environmental factors

Attention must be given to the environment to ensure there is sufficient room for the resident to manoeuvre with their chosen walking appliance. Safe mobility requires an appreciation of one's limitations and of environmental hazards (Vassallo *et al.*, 2004).

■ **Visibility**

Wheelchairs and scooters lower the mid-range of vision of the user, causing difficulty for users to see the route ahead. ODPM (2006) provides clear guidance on the design of external and internal doors. All doors should have vision panels so that other people who are approaching can be clearly seen. If there is a large area of glass, for example a patio door or large window, residents with impaired vision may bump into glass areas and bruise themselves or fall. To avoid inadvertent human contact the glass should have 'manifestation' which contrasts with the background. Traditional acid etching or sandblasted areas produced before installation, or simply an opaque film applied to the glass, can achieve sufficient manifestation. Dots, squares, stripes or bespoke designs can be used. The regulations suggest that a logo or signs of 150 mm or continuous bands be used. There should be two bands, 50 mm in width, at 850 mm to 1000 mm and 1400 mm to 1600 mm from floor level.

■ **Trip hazards**

Small doormats and rugs are particularly hazardous and should be avoided. Several retailers sell doormats with a sloping rubberised edge that facilitates the passage of wheeled appliances. Spillages should be cleared and wet floors identified by adequate signage.

■ **Safe storage**

All appliances should be stored safely and not pose a fall hazard. Some homes have designated space for wheelchairs and walking frame storage. To protect the walls the surfaces can be covered with clear Perspex.

Observing changes and providing feedback

Residents should be given feedback when mobilising. It is important to correct postural and gait problems before they develop into bad habits. Poor gait can be due to the wearing of non-supportive footwear and will require addressing. It is important to record changes and speak to appropriate people (other carers, line managers, GP, nurses and therapists) if mobility deteriorates. Alteration of medication, exercises or a more supportive (or less supportive) walking aid may be indicated. Inter-professional collaboration is important to ensure the optimum level of mobility and safety.

Conclusion

Maintaining mobility in life is essential to remain independent and to live full and satisfying lives for as long as possible. It is vital that care staff provide support to help residents re-mobilise and thereafter maintain their mobility. With advancing age and disability it can be difficult to maintain a good level of mobility. Mobility can be encouraged in many ways by providing active support to a resident to maintain their level of mobility. Staff can allow residents to do as much of an activity as possible for themselves or to undertake recreational activities that encourage a good range of movement.

Key points

- Mobility is a complex function that can become impaired through ageing, disability or lack of exercise.
- Encourage residents to keep as mobile as possible.
- Correct bad posture and compensatory patterns of movements.
- Pay attention to environmental influences and ensure that good housekeeping policies are followed.
- Provide feedback to residents and other staff involved.

CHAPTER 23

Mobility appliances

Advances in technology have facilitated the development of lightweight yet stronger walking appliances. There are many different forms of walking appliance, giving more choice to the consumer, and there is an extensive choice of outlets in which they can be purchased.

Main types of walking appliance

Although walking appliances help to steady and reduce weight bearing on lower limb joints, they cannot erase balance difficulties completely. The size of the base of support affects the stability provided; for example, a walking stick will not give as much stability as a walking frame.

■ **Walking sticks**

Sticks are used to give slight support and to help with balance. These are no longer simply wooden sticks with straight or curved handles. Many sticks have shaped handgrips which are useful for people with a limited range of hand movements or when gripping is uncomfortable, perhaps due to rheumatoid arthritis. Some sticks have clip-on attachments that enable the stick to be hooked over the edge of a table. Leather wrist straps enable sticks to be looped over the arm when negotiating a series of steps if a two-handed grip is needed on supportive rails. Adjustable height sticks can be obtained and some fold up to be carried in a bag to be used only when needed. Some walking sticks, including folding sticks, have integral seats that are useful if the user tires or becomes short of breath. Two sticks (or crutches) may be necessary, but the four-point walking pattern (stick, leg, stick, leg) may be difficult for a resident to learn and a walking frame may be easier to manage.

■ **Tripods and quadrupods**

These are basically a stick with three (tripod) or four (quadrupod) legs. They provide greater stability and will 'stand up' when not in use without falling over. They do not seem to be issued as commonly as in the past, perhaps due to the introduction of other ranges of walking appliances.

■ **Crutches**

There are several types of crutches, e.g. elbow crutches, gutter crutches, axilla crutches and Canadian crutches (these have a padded ring that circles the arm). Most of these are adjustable in height.

■ **Walking frames**

A walking frame provides more support than a stick. Walking frames should not be used as a means of rising but only held when a standing posture is achieved, unless they are specially designed. Several variations are available, e.g. folding frames, triangular shaped frames (these are useful in confined spaces), padded forearm supports (high walkers) and ones with wheels (rollators).

Alkjær *et al.* (2006) identified that the walking pattern of healthy people using a rollator was characterised by increased hip flexion, decreased ankle dorsiflexion and knee flexion. This reduced the ankle and the knee joint moments significantly and the movement produced by the hip extensors was increased. As several of these muscle groups are used to stand and sit, to maintain posture, and for trunk control, it is important to ensure that other forms of activity are carried out to maintain the underused muscle groups. This can be achieved via a structured activity programme.

■ **Household trolleys**

Trolleys can be used as walking appliances and some have handlebar types of handgrip for added stability. Trolleys should be the correct height for the individual resident. The advantage of a trolley is that it can help transport items from room to room, as well as giving some support.

■ **Manual wheelchairs**

Wheelchairs within the home are either ones that are used to transport the resident (transit or attendant wheelchair) or that residents can propel themselves (self-propelling wheelchair). Transit wheelchairs have smaller wider wheels and provide a more comfortable ride. Self-propelling wheelchairs have two large wheels (normally the two back wheels). The larger wheels have an inner ring or an inner capstan wheel to enable the resident to push. Some wheelchairs have two inner rings on one side to enable operation by one hand.

■ **Powered wheelchairs**

These can be supplied from the wheelchair centre or perhaps the resident may have purchased one before admission. It is important to carry out a risk assessment to ensure that the resident is able to use the wheelchair safely without danger to themselves or others. Some powered wheelchairs are only suitable for indoor use. Features on outdoor models can include kerb climbers, variable speeds, canopies, capes, lights and indicators. Residents may prefer a powered three- or four-wheeled scooter to use outdoors.

Carrying items when using a walking appliance

Transporting items around can pose problems when using a walking aid. The simplest method is to use a shoulder bag. If a walking frame or rollator is used a carrier bag can be attached. Several retailers sell bags and trays that attach to the frame, or 'home-made' bags can be used.

Correct adjustments of mobility appliances

Many walking appliances are adjustable in height. It is important to ensure they are the correct height, yet often they are not. If walking aids are too low the walking pattern will be impaired, causing stopped posture or backache. If the appliance is too high it will not provide sufficient support when walking.

- **Stick, tripods, quadrupods, walkers, elbow crutches and trolleys**
As a general rule the handle should be level with the wrist when the arm is held at the side, or level with the hip joint. This provides a slightly flexed arm position when weight bearing, yet allows for the arm carrying the mobility appliance to comfortably bring the appliance in front, without over-balancing, maintaining an erect posture.

- **Axilla crutch**
There should be around three finger widths of space between the top of an axilla crutch and the armpit.

- **Wheelchairs**
A wheelchair is rarely adjusted to an individual if it is delivered straight from the wheelchair centre or supplier. It is important therefore to check each new appliance to ensure that it is appropriate for an individual. The footplates often need adjusting so that when the individual is sat on the seat, perhaps on a wheelchair cushion, the thighs are parallel to the ground.

Further information on mobility equipment

The Disabled Living Foundation has several factsheets on mobility equipment (http://www.dlf.org.uk/public/factsheets.html):

- Choosing walking equipment
- Choosing a powered wheelchair
- Choosing a scooter or buggy
- Choosing a standard self-propelling wheelchair
- Choosing an active user wheelchair
- Choosing an attendant propelled wheelchair
- Out and about with your wheelchair

Care of appliances

All appliances should be cleaned and checked regularly as part of a maintenance programme.

■ Walking appliances
Sticks, crutches and walkers have a slip-resistant ending or a rubber ferrule. Ferrules require replacing and they are not all the same size. Chemists often carry a stock of ferrules and they can be obtained from larger equipment suppliers.

■ Orthotics
Appliances such as splints, callipers, foot-drop splints and collars should be inspected regularly. Ensure that the appliances fit properly and do not rub or cause pressure areas.

■ Wheelchairs
To avoid mismatching, all detachable parts can be labelled or colour coded.

Wheelchairs should be checked to ensure that they are working properly. Moving parts should be oiled. Sometimes the brakes can work loose and a nut may need tightening. A tiny tear in the seat of wheelchair can easily tear across with the weight of a resident.

Although the local wheelchair centre deals with repair of wheelchairs provided free to individuals, day-to-day care is the responsibility of the home. If the chair belongs to a resident there may be a residual warranty on the wheelchair to cover maintenance, replacement of parts and repair. Storage facilities will need to be provided and battery-powered chairs will need recharging.

Observing changes

Some alterations in an individual's mobility are not due purely to medical or structural bodily changes, but to compensatory patterns of movement and bad habits. Examples of this are stooped or slouched posture, tendency to stand on one leg and poor sitting posture. Bad postural habits can lead to weakness of muscle groups due to insufficient use. This in turn causes more dependency on the stronger muscles, with further weakening of the muscles that are not being used, often resulting in an abnormal gait (walking pattern). Weaver (2005) discusses functional problems that may occur and need reporting, e.g. transferring problems, swaying and staggering. It is important not only to observe and record changes in mobility and to provide feedback, but also to try to ascertain the reasons for the change. Medication can cause adverse effects and affect the initiation of movement patterns.

Risk assessment and feedback

Risk assessments should include how the resident mobilises within the care home. Take special note if there are ramps or steps within the home, particularly outside the resident's room, or if a ground floor bedroom has patio access that does not lead into a secured area. Falls are common in older people, and although hip protectors can help to cushion falls they do not necessarily prevent fractures occurring.

Several residents may have self-purchased walking appliances without any professional guidance and the appliance may be the wrong height or not suited to their needs. If the walking appliance seems unsuitable refer this to a physiotherapist or occupational therapist, as they can advise on suitability.

Physiotherapists will assist in identifying problem areas and devising a programme of exercises to help correct abnormal patterns of movement and improve coordination and strength. Movement patterns may need to be re-learned and it is essential that practice is provided in between sessions. Care staff have a vital role to encourage any prescribed exercises.

Problems with mobility affect the way an individual moves when performing activities. Occupational therapists can help work out if using a different technique is required or an assistive device is needed. They can also help advise on activities for care staff to incorporate into an activities programme that are within a resident's capabilities, e.g. activities to improve coordination or muscle strength. Movement patterns can be used in a structured movement to music programme as described in Chapter 24. Occupational therapists can also advise the home on ways to facilitate mobility and to make the environment easier for residents with physical problems to cope in, and to prevent falls.

Medical and orthopaedic involvement may be necessary to resolve many of the problems, but help may also be needed to gently encourage movement. It is important to record the level of mobility that a resident has and to note any changes in this to the appropriate person so that it can be dealt with effectively.

Conclusion

All staff have a vital role in supporting residents to maintain their level of mobility. Observation of changes should be communicated to appropriate people involved in the care of a resident. Attention to good housekeeping of the immediate environment and regular checks on mobility appliances is needed. Care staff can take many steps to ensure that residents are safe when using appliances. Maintaining mobility is crucial within a care environment and encompasses all aspects of personal care, recreation and general mobility.

Key points

- Many types of walking appliance are available.
- It is essential that residents who rely on walking aids have the most suitable one for their needs.
- Keep the walking equipment well maintained.
- Risk assessments should be undertaken that include environmental factors.
- Report any changes in mobility to appropriate staff.

Movement to music

Moving to music is a popular leisure activity that ranges from simply tapping fingers or feet in time to music to energetic dancing. People gain pleasure from participation, regardless of their standard of performance.

Benefits of movement to music

People living in a care environment can benefit from this activity in many ways:

- It is an enjoyable social activity.
- It provides a safe and effective way to exercise specific muscle groups; improve energy levels and stamina; improve suppleness, coordination and speed of movement; and increase muscle strength.
- Rehabilitation aims are reinforced by targeting specific problem areas, such as general weakness or postural and mobility problems.
- Metabolic rate is increased, thereby reducing body fat and weight and helping to lower cholesterol.
- Cardiovascular efficiency and circulation are improved.
- Sleep patterns are improved, particularly if relaxation is taught and reinforced at bedtime.

Although a resident may become frailer, it is vital to encourage maximum mobility. Deterioration in physical ability leads to an increase in dependence on others for daily living activities. The saying 'use it or lose it' also applies to people in care.

Factors to consider

The culture of the home should be conducive to carrying out movement to music. It is important to have a good team of staff and a hazard-free environment, and to know your residents' capabilities.

Team of staff

Managers should involve residents and staff in recreational sessions and encourage a proactive atmosphere. With a supportive team, individuals can play to their strengths. Staff that do not take the movement to music session can help by:

- 'Brainstorming' ideas for the sessions
- Finding suitable music or planning movement patterns and routines
- Moving residents into the room to be used and helping them during the session
- Being 'on call' for toileting – it is impossible to carry out a session when dual duties are needed
- Helping make items to use in sessions (see 'Props' below)

A conducive environment

A well-ventilated warm room should be selected, with suitable seating that allows sufficient space for arm and leg movements. Some wheelchairs may tip when occupants lean too far forwards, so wheelchair users should be transferred into suitable seating. Alternatively, footplates can be removed and the client's feet placed on the floor, raising the feet if necessary.

Know your residents' capabilities and limitations

The clients' medical problems and any 'hidden' conditions must be known. Risk assessments should be checked, remembering that changes can occur quickly with a resident's medical condition.

Consider the aims of the session

Gentle exercising and stretches should be provided to maintain suppleness, strength, coordination and range of movement. Visiting therapists will have specific guidelines for residents. Movement patterns should be included within the sessions, to maximise the therapist's input and provide more opportunities for therapeutic movements.

Choice of music

Music often holds special meanings, triggering memories of joy or sadness. Wenborn (2003) explains the value of music within care homes. The music chosen should be enjoyable and appropriate to the group. Residents can be asked which singers or songs they like. If language or memory is a problem, then ask the resident's relatives or friends.

Planning the session

The following basic points must first be considered:

1. Decide on the number of residents.
2. Choose a suitable room.
3. Decide on the length of the session (from 20–60 minutes) and time of day.
4. Do not let clients exercise on a full stomach, e.g. directly after lunch.
5. Select music with a regular beat.
6. Work out the movements or exercises to specific tracks.
7. Arrange for additional help if needed.
8. Check that any equipment you need is in working order.
9. Ensure residents are fit to participate (agree actions with care plan).
10. Ensure that loose-fitting clothing is worn and that residents' dignity is preserved.

Movements should be paced to suit the residents, with emphasis placed on correct breathing and slow, unrushed movements. The session should start with a warm up, followed by upper body movements and lower body movements, and finish with a 'cool down' session, using a different track of music for each. This should last for about 20 minutes.

How do you start the session?

Staff should take into account any barriers to communication, such as deafness, sight defects, understanding problems and language difficulties. Residents with communication problems should be seated nearby and the use of communication aids, such as spectacles and hearing aids, should be encouraged. The 'activity organiser' taking the session should explain what he, or she, is doing and why. If participants feel dizzy or tired, it should be stressed that they must stop and rest; particularly with people who have not exercised recently. A little additional movement is better than nothing at all.

Warming up

The session should start with gentle 'warm-up' movements to loosen and stretch the muscles. Use one or two tracks of the music, taking each muscle group through its maximum range of movement.

Anderson (2000) describes stretches from a seated position and advises on the importance of taking activity slowly, raising the body temperature to a level where injury is less likely. Most 'keep fit' books include warm ups that can be adapted for seated users, such as:

- Arms stretched up above the head, down to the shoulders and then onto the lap.
- Slumping in the chair, then straightening up.
- Bending the legs under the chair or wheelchair.

As a general rule, inhale when arms are elevated or when shoulders are drawn back and exhale on forward or downward movements. To encourage full use of lung capacity, deep breathing exercises can be included.

During the session

The activity organiser needs to decide whether to do 'pure movements' or 'activity-based movements'.

■ Pure movement

In pure movement, one should aim for a mid-range of movement, gradually increasing the range. A leg or back movement could be alternated with a hand or arm movement. The exercise should fit the music; for example, faster music for hands and legs and slower music for back, shoulders and head. Bilateral arm movements can be used with people suffering from hemiparesis (partial paralysis of one side of the body). To improve hand coordination and grip strength, hand exercises can be incorporated.

Complicated movement routines should not be tried, as these are difficult to learn.

■ Activity-based movement

Activity-based movements are based on well-known activities, such as playing the piano, swimming and tug-of-war. Examples of diagrammatic sequences of actions carried out while seated are provided by Graham (2000) and include 'directing traffic' and 'rag doll'. Quarta (2001) provides a seated exercise programme. Songs that specify actions, such as 'I am the music man', 'Knees up Mother Brown' and 'Lambeth walk', can be tried. Dance routines such as the 'Hokey Cokey' and 'Macarena' can be adapted to the sitting position. Inspiration can be found in the movement patterns of Tai Chi.

Stretches

Stretches can be used within a movement-to-music session to improve flexibility. Stretches are achieved in comfortable supportive positions held with muscles feeling slight tension, not extreme tension. Rapid body movements are not recommended, as this can cause muscle tearing and ligament damage, with a resultant reduction of joint stability. Books on yoga, such as by Lalvani (2000), describe stretches in more detail.

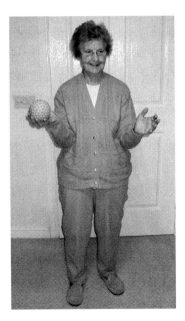

Grasp and release using 'props' (© Julie Swann 2007).

Props

A variety of props can be used to exercise with. These can be everyday items, for example:

- Scarves, to encourage wide-sweeping arm movements.
- Soft balls/pompoms, transferred from hand to hand with emphasis on grasp and release.
- Walking sticks, for upper limb and trunk control.

As the session progresses...

Staff should encourage and provide feedback to residents through verbal and non-verbal methods, such as nods, smiles, facial expressions and gestures. It is vital to ensure that residents are doing exercises correctly and safely. Help should be provided when needed, particularly to facilitate active range of movement. Staff should be prepared to alter either the music or the movements.

At the end of the session

One music track of cool-down movements should be done to restore the body system to a pre-exercise level. Otherwise the muscles may shorten, causing stiffness, cramp or pain the following day. Large movements grading down to smaller, slower movements are recommended.

A long session should be ended with 5–15 minutes of systemic relaxation, to wind down. Relaxation is described in Chapter 20. It is also termed visualisation or cognitive quieting and is used after yoga or pilates. Graham (2000) outlines a systemic relaxation session.

During relaxation, residents should be asked to sit comfortably with their hands on their laps and be encouraged to take some slow, deep breaths. Residents should be guided through systemically tensing each muscle group, then relaxing. The activity organiser can describe a restful scene, such as quiet woodland, a trickling stream or a deserted beach. A track (or several) of gentle instrumental music can be played. When the music finishes, encourage participants to stretch out their arms and then their legs, curl their spines and uncurl, and then relax.

After the session

Residents should be asked for feedback on the session. Further activities can be included within the residents' weekly programme to encourage maximum use of their abilities.

There may be a standard format for recording activities, but if not, short records should be kept as an *aide mémoire*. The names of participants, music and type of movements used should be noted. Any adverse effects should also be noted, and any problems promptly reported to senior staff.

Further resources

Books on fitness for the older and frail person are available from local libraries and bookshops or via the Internet. Exercises from them can be adapted to the sitting position or 'toned down'.

Physiotherapists, local clinics and hospitals will provide guidelines on exercise for specific conditions. Body posture can be corrected through re-education of resting, sitting and walking posture, using for example the Alexandra technique.

Conclusion

Movement to music is a low-cost, enjoyable activity that can be used in many care settings. It should be a light-hearted, fun and pleasurable social activity. It is important to build up slowly, so activity should start with gentle, slow movements. The choice of music sets the mood for the session and may develop into a 'sing-along'. Movement to music is easier to carry out and more enjoyable if the main part is action-related. It becomes easier with practice – which applies to both the recipient and the provider.

Key points

- Movement to music encourages social interaction.
- Benefits include improvements in physical, psychological and cognitive abilities.
- Development of an individual's maximum range of movement is important.
- A resident's medical conditions must be known to ensure awareness of contra-indications and incorporation of beneficial movement patterns.
- Movement to music is a low-cost activity that can be included in a recreational or rehabilitation programme.

PART 10

Major disabilities and ways of minimising problems

CHAPTER 25

Understanding and reducing the risk of a stroke

On average, around 25% of care home residents will have suffered from a stroke. The chance of someone who is over the age of 85 years having a stroke is 100 times greater than that of a person who is aged 35–45 years (Kwan, 2001). Given that the age profile of the UK population is rising, it is understandable that there is a national drive to reduce the number of incidents of coronary heart disease and strokes (Department of Health, 1999).

> In the next hour, 12 people in the UK will have a stroke. Four of those people will recover, four will have permanent disabilities and four will die. (The Stroke Association, 2005)

In so-called developed countries, strokes are the third most common cause of death. It is the commonest cause of adult disability in the UK, with 130,000 people each year having a stroke (Rudd *et al.*, 2000). World Health Organization data indicates that 4.5 million people die each year from stroke (Perkins, 2002). The Intercollegiate Stroke Working Party's (2004) *National Clinical Guidelines for Stroke* provides more information on this disease. In autumn 2005, the Stroke Association launched a *Stroke is a Medical Emergency* campaign to raise awareness of warning signs of a stroke.

It is important that people suffering a stroke receive diagnosis and treatment as soon as possible after the first symptoms. Although the following chapters focus on people with a stroke, many of the approaches are equally beneficial to people whose problems affect mobility and upper limb function.

What is a stroke?

Strokes are not a new disease. Ancient Greeks believed that if someone suffered a stroke (or any sudden incapacity), the gods had struck them down (MedicineNet, 2006). Apoplexy, cerebrovascular accident and cerebrovasuclar events are all terms used to describe a stroke. 'Apoplexy' is Greek for 'seizure' and 'plexia' is Greek for 'a stroke'.

What causes a stroke?

Strokes result from an impaired blood supply to a part of the brain. Onset can be sudden or gradual, causing temporary or permanent loss of function to part of the brain affected. Strokes vary greatly in severity depending on the location of the area of the brain that is affected, the extent of the impairment of blood supply and the degree of collateral blood supply.

Strokes do not only affect older people; babies and young people have them, often as a result of a thrombosis (formation of a blood clot) or a haemorrhage (due to abnormality of blood vessels in the brain). Most stroke victims have warning signs that go unheeded (Table 25.1). It is vital to find out the cause so correct treatment can be prescribed.

There are two broad types of stroke (Rudd *et al.*, 2000):

- **Cerebral haemorrhage** (around 20% of strokes):
A bleed can occur after a fall or a sudden rupture of an artery (aneurysm), causing bleeding into or around the brain

- **Cerebral thrombosis/embolism** (around 80% of strokes):
A blood clot or plaque, perhaps from another part of the body, that causes blockage of blood vessels in the brain.

Mild transient ischaemic attacks (TIAs), termed 'mini-strokes', can result from a small thrombosis or emboli (tissue fragment that can obstruct blood flow). A TIA can result from clots dislodging and travelling to the brain, or from weak cardiac walls, cumulating in reduced cardiac output. The symptoms resolve in 24 hours (Rudd *et al.*, 2000). However, the risk of developing a stroke after a hemispheric TIA can be as high as 20% within the first month, with the greatest risk within the first 72 hours (Intercollegiate Stroke Working Party, 2004). A TIA should be viewed as a warning of an impending, more severe or permanently disabling stroke and immediate medical assessment is urgently needed to ascertain the underlying cause.

Table 25.1 Warning signs of a stroke (Stanford Stroke Center, 2006)

- Sudden weakness, numbness or paralysis of the face, arm or leg (especially on one side of the body).
- Loss of speech or trouble talking or understanding language.
- Sudden loss of vision, particularly in only one eye.
- Sudden, severe headache with no apparent cause.
- Unexplained dizziness, loss of balance or coordination (especially if associated with any of the above symptoms).

Head injury, encephalitis, cerebral tumours, cerebral abscess and multiple sclerosis can also cause symptoms similar to those produced by a stroke.

Effects of stroke

'Silent' strokes or mild TIAs can go unnoticed; others cause only a short period of muscle weakness. A severe stroke can cause loss of most movement patterns down one side of the body and sensory problems, but most stroke sufferers have some return of movement and abilities. Complete loss of function down one side is termed hemiplegia, and partial loss of movement is termed hemiparesis. Even with a mild stroke, a loss of physical function may cause problems with daily life. Speech, balance, perceptual and visual problems may occur. Table 25.2 shows the effects of a stroke.

Complications of a stroke

The physical consequences of neurological dysfunction caused by a stroke can be made worse by spasticity (increase in muscle tone) and compensatory movement patterns. Both these problems are discussed in Chapter 26. Complications arising from a stroke can include shoulder problems, oedematous hands, contractures (soft tissue shortening) and respiratory problems. Sensory and psychological problems car also arise. Severe strokes can lead to unconsciousness, difficulty breathing and even death. The incidence of another stroke within five years of a first stroke is 30–43% (Mant *et al.*, 2004), so it is equally important to help prevent its recurrence.

Risk factors

Several risk factors for stroke are unevenly spread across society. People with limited income are often exposed to the highest risks. Certain stroke risk factors are beyond control, for example being male or over the age of 55 years, or having a family history of stroke. Afro-Caribbean and South Asian people are more likely to suffer a stroke than Europeans (Rudd *et al.*, 2000). Stanford Stroke Center (2006) has an online stroke risk assessment test (http:// strokecenter.stanford.edu/consent.html).

Table 25.2 What does the brain do? (Patricia Neal Rehabilitation Center, 2005)

Left hemisphere (Stroke on left side) Right side of body affected	Right hemisphere (Stroke on right side) Left side of body affected
Motor speech	Attention span
Expressive speech	Impulse control
Movement on right side of body	Movement on left side of body
Emotion Control	Initiates activities you want to do
Writing	Remembering visual objects
Locating body in space	Recognition of faces
Understanding mathematics	Drawing skills
Reading numbers and letters	Awareness of the left side of the body
Recognising objects	Emotional stability
Remembering written information	Measuring distances of objects to body

Lifestyle risk factors

Several of the preventive measures for stroke are similar to those for obesity, secondary onset diabetes and heart disease. Some risk factors are interrelated, such as obesity and physical inactivity. Other risk factors are:

- Poor nutrition due to consuming too much fat and salt and insufficient fruit and vegetables
- High blood pressure
- High LDL (low-density lipoprotein) cholesterol levels
- Excess alcohol intake
- Smoking (Perkins, 2002)

Stroke prevention

Humans are not biologically designed to live on high-fat diets or to smoke or drink excessively, and cardiovascular systems pay the price of over-indulgence. Many medical risk factors can be controlled, such as diabetes, high cholesterol, arterial hypertension (high blood pressure), migraine, heart and circulatory disease. Drugs like aspirin or warfarin help to reduce the risks of thrombosis and strokes. Balanced menus, weight control, regular exercise, regular checks of blood pressure, reduction of smoking, alcohol, caffeine and salt, and control of diabetes are considered below.

■ Balanced menus

In 2004 the Stroke Awareness Week launched the *Eat a Rainbow – Beat a Stroke* campaign. The aim was to encourage healthier eating by highlighting the benefits of eating five portions of fruit a day. Ideally diets should be low in fats, especially saturated fatty acids, and low in cholesterol. There are two sorts of cholesterol: 'good' high-density lipoprotein (HDL) and 'bad' low-density lipoprotein (LDL). LDL-cholesterol level can be lowered by eating a low-fat diet and, if required, by taking medication. Exercising can raise HDL cholesterol level. The ideal blood cholesterol level is less than 5 mmol/l. Statins can reduce cholesterol level (Collins, 2005) by blocking enzymes needed for cholesterol, mainly in the liver. The main statins (with brand names) are: atorvastatin (Lipitor), fluvastatin (Lescol), pravastatin (Lipostat), rosuvastatin (Crestor) and simvastatin (Zocor, Zocor Heart-Pro, Simzal) (NHS Direct, 2006b).

■ Weight control

Ensuring that residents have a balanced diet and encouraging mobility and independence can achieve this.

■ Regular exercise

Gentle exercise several times a week can help control weight and improve circulation. By reducing weight, the risk of high blood pressure, heart disease and adult-onset (type 2) diabetes decreases.

■ Monitoring blood pressure

Regular blood pressure checks are important as high blood pressure causes 40% of all strokes in the UK (The Stroke Association, 2005). Adults' normal blood pressure is around 120/80 and a blood pressure over 140/90 is considered high. Smoking, obesity, lack of exercise and stress can all raise blood pressure. Lowering blood pressure even by 5–6 mmHg (Perkins, 2002) reduces the risk of both stroke and heart disease.

■ Reducing smoking

Smoking increases the heart rate and raises blood pressure. It causes increased 'stickiness' between blood platelets, which can cause thrombosis. Post mortem examinations on smokers show more atherosclerosis than those on non-smokers. Although it is perhaps unrealistic to expect elderly people to stop smoking, residents may choose to reduce their consumption of cigarettes.

■ **Reducing alcohol intake**

'Binge drinkers' are twice as likely to have a stroke compared to non-drinkers (The Stroke Association, 2005) and alcoholic drinks should be reduced to two drinks a day.

■ **Reducing caffeine and salt intake**

Caffeine intake should be reduced to four cups a day and salt to less than 3 g a day. This can help to reduce high blood pressure (MedicineNet, 2005).

■ **Controlling diabetes**

Untreated diabetes can damage blood vessels throughout the body and lead to atherosclerosis.

Medical management and medication

Preventative medication falls into two major categories: anticoagulants (such as warfarin or ximelgatran) and antiplatelet agents (such as aspirin, dipyridamole and clopidogrel). Acute medical management of a stroke depends on the cause. Medication to 'thin blood' and 'clot-busting' drugs could save the life of someone with ischaemic stroke, but may worsen the condition of someone suffering haemorrhagic stroke. Wiebers (2001) comments: 'To put it bluntly, you don't fix a clogged pipe the same way you fix a leaky one'.

Botox (botulinum toxin) can be given as an injection and is gaining popularity in the treatment of contractures. It works by blocking the action of nerves on muscles, reducing stiffness. It can take 2–3 days to take effect and lasts 4–6 months. Muscular relaxants can help when spasticity is a problem, but most medication has side effects, including drowsiness, dizziness and dry mouth.

Conclusion

Most care homes have residents who have suffered from a stroke. Care staff can help in the prevention of strokes by encouraging residents to have a healthy lifestyle. There are many practical ways that care staff can help facilitate the return of function and increase their resident's level of abilities and independence. These will be discussed in the following chapters.

Key points

- A stroke is generally caused by blockage of blood flow to the brain, or rupture of an artery.
- Sudden tingling, weakness or paralysis on one side of the body or difficulty with balance, speaking, swallowing or vision can be symptoms of a stroke.
- Stroke prevention involves reducing risk factors like high blood pressure, raised cholesterol and smoking.
- Healthy diets and exercise should be encouraged.
- Risk factors for strokes and heart disease are similar.

CHAPTER 26

Strokes – what can care staff do?

Some people may not be admitted into hospital after a stroke, particularly if no surgical intervention is anticipated. After a stroke, early gradual mobilisation is important. Although some care homes have their own rehabilitation staff, many do not. There is a great deal that care staff can do to facilitate recovery and prevent abnormal movement patterns and other disabling symptoms developing. Even several years after a stroke, if a resident has any residual effects stemming from a stroke, further rehabilitation can help.

The physical signs of neurological dysfunction caused by a stroke are weakness or loss of active movement. Complications like spasticity (increase in muscle tone), compensatory abnormal movement patterns, contractures (tight muscle tendons) and shoulder pain all add to functional loss of movement. In the longer term these complications will adversely affect abilities.

Principles of treatment

Therapists aim to reduce and prevent stroke-related complications and abnormal movement patterns. Often, this is achieved by reducing the compensatory patterns of movement and muscle tone that causes tightness in muscle groups. Correcting any abnormal patterns of compensatory movements is important, and this will be concentrated on in the initial part of any physical therapy.

Several residents who have had a stoke may have a typical 'hemiplegic pattern' of movement (Table 26.1). The upper limb muscles tighten as a result of spasticity in a flexor pattern of movement. Spasticity can lead to contractures. The hand is often clenched and the fingers can dig into the palm of the hand. The stronger anti-gravity muscles (extensor muscles) in the legs can tighten and tend to show a greater degree of spasticity.

Table 26.1 Typical pattern of spasticity.

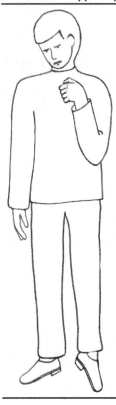

- The head is flexed to the affected side and rotated to the unaffected side.

- The shoulder is depressed and pulled forwards.

- The arm is held against the body and medially rotated.

- The elbow is flexed.

- The forearm is pronated with the thumb towards the centre line of the body.

- The wrist is flexed and pulled towards the little finger side (ulnar deviated).

- The fingers are flexed into the palm.

- The trunk is side-flexed on the affected side.

- The pelvis is pulled upwards and backwards.

- The hip is laterally rotated.

- The leg is either flexed and abducted or extended and adducted.

- The foot is plantar flexed and inverted.

Image by Angela Munslow 2006.

What can care staff do to help?

If the home has any therapists or visiting therapists, it is important for care staff to observe activities. Movement patterns can be carried out, under supervision, between therapists' visits. Care staff can also help residents by assisting with the organisation of tasks, including pacing and timing of activities.

Positioning

Initially in a severe stroke (dense hemiplegia), there may be a period during which there is no perceivable muscle tone (flaccid hemiplegia) in an arm and leg. Sometimes only the arm or leg will be affected. If a loss of function occurred, it is important that correct positioning is carried out to avoid abnor-

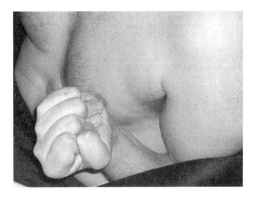

Increase in muscle tone (spasticity) (© Julie Swann 2007).

mal movement patterns developing. Even touching and moving the affected side can trigger spasticity unless slow smooth movements are used. Additional pillows can support flaccid limbs and care staff can help by using correct positioning techniques. In addition to supporting an affected arm when sitting or lying, the arm should also be supported when a wheelchair is used.

Avoiding shoulder problems

The shoulder joint is described as a 'loose lax' structure (rather like an old elastic corset that has been 'in the wash' too many times). The shoulder muscles and ligaments keep the head of the humerus in the ball and socket joint. If the muscles are weak and the arm is not supported, subluxation (partial dislocation) can occur. This can lead to a 'frozen shoulder', caused by the weight of the arm pulling on the capsule and ligaments. Pulling on the affected arm (or any other joint) should be avoided when moving the resident, as this can damage the shoulder joint. Whenever possible, the arm should be rested outstretched on a pillow with the shoulder joint supported and the hand in supination (palm turned up) if possible.

Bilateral arm exercises

If the resident is sitting in a chair, ensure that both feet are on the ground, about 9–12 inches apart, with the resident weightbearing equally through the buttocks. The following basic exercises are useful if there are coordination problems, and will help to develop trunk control and 'core stability'. If the affected arm is flaccid (no tone), try to encourage bilateral arm exercises with the fingers entwined and the affected thumb on the top:

■ Lift up the arms towards the ceiling.
■ Push the arms forwards and straighten the elbows.
■ Lift the arms up, then stretch out to the unaffected side, then the affected side.

The emphasis should be on the pushing forwards and the arms should be slowly brought back towards the body. This is so that the extensor pattern of movement is strengthened, rather than encouraging the 'typical hemi' posture (Table 26.1) of a flexed upper limb spasticity in the arm, although not all people present with spasticity. Exercises can be carried out when the resident is in bed.

Preventing contractures

All the joints of affected limbs should be passively moved through a full range of movement, at least once daily. This can be incorporated in activities. It is vital to avoid contractures developing in the tendons. Staff can encourage the use of bilateral arm exercises encouraging limbs to be taken through a partial range of movement. Some occupational therapists use hand splints in a 'tone-normalising' position to prevent contractures. Medication can reduce the effect of spasticity but has side effects.

Application of ice to reduce spasticity

By applying an ice cube directly onto the back of the hand (the muscle belly), the hand often loosens, particularly if the thumb is gently pulled away first. If there is oedema then exercises can help to reduce this and advice should be sought from a physiotherapist.

Preventing foot drop

If the foot is not positioned correctly, contractures and foot drop may occur (see Table 26.1). Foot drop is caused when there is difficulty or failure to lift the front part of the foot due to muscle weakness. Tightening of the Achilles tendon caused by spasticity can also cause foot drop that will impede development of a good walking pattern. To help reduce spasticity and stretch the Achilles tendon, the affected foot should be positioned flat on the floor and weight put though this when the resident is sitting, and also when standing. It is important not to place a board or pillow against the foot as this can increase spasticity. Untreated foot drop can lead to shortening (contracture) of the Achilles tendon and, when walking, weight will only be taken through the front part of the foot (Table 26.1).

Basic care

Some basic personal care activities will be required; for example, ensuring that bed-bound residents are turned every 6 hours to prevent pressure areas from forming. Special pressure-relieving mattresses and chair cushions can be obtained. Oral care is important, particularly if liquids are not allowed by mouth due to problems swallowing. To avoid dryness, soreness or infection, Rudd *et al.* (2000) describe keeping the mouth moist by using mouthwash, wet wipes, Vaseline on the lips, giving ice cubes to suck, and ensuring that dentures are clean. Muscle tone in the hand may decrease when a limb or the body is immersed in warm water, whereas being uncomfortable, exposed to cold, exerting effort, fatigue or raised emotion may increase the muscle tone. Therapists can assist with suitable activity planning.

Assisting with mobilisation

Once a resident's medical condition is stabilised, tasks like turning from side to side and self-care activities (feeding, grooming and dressing) should be encouraged. It is important for correct, normal patterns of movement to be carried out. Unfortunately, people who are not treated by a therapist may develop abnormal patterns of movement (Table 26.2).

Movement must be experienced for recovery to take place. It is important to regain trunk control before walking is started. A wide base of support (such as a reclining chair or bed) will reduce spasticity; conversely, a narrow base of support (such as perching or standing) increases spasticity. If a narrower (less) base of support is applied then muscle tone can be positively increased in a flaccid limb.

By using re-education movement patterns and techniques to reduce spasticity (for example weight bearing through a limb), this pattern of movement can be minimised. This is one of the principles behind 'normal movement', a technique that evolved from Bobath (1990) (refer to Chapter 33).

If a person feels insecure, tired, generally unwell, emotional or stressed, or has perceptual problems, muscle tone and mobility can all be affected. Taking pauses and only carrying out tasks when the resident has energy will help.

Problems with effort

Unfortunately, effort can make the arm go into a flexor pattern again. Interlinking the hands and encouraging forward movement can also help reduce this tightening. *Do not*:

- Encourage gripping of objects, as this will only increase spasticity. Concentrate on slow grasp and release.
- Place a ball or other object into the palm of the affected arm. This will stimulate the palm of the hand and increase spasticity.
- Leave the resident sitting in a chair without ensuring that the shoulder joint is well supported.
- Put the affected arm into a static sling all of the time as this may increase spasticity and contractures. However, a subluxed shoulder may need some support.

Visual and perceptual problems

As hemianopia (loss of half the visual field) is common, check that residents have a full range of vision. Staff should also observe for any signs of visual neglect and encourage the resident to cross the 'midline' by deliberately placing items in the neglected range of vision, speaking to the resident from the affected side, placing a table and drinks on the affected side. As improvement occurs tasks can then be carried out beyond the mid-line.

If a stroke affects the left side, perceptual problems and visual neglect may occur. Residents may not know how to use an everyday item (dyspraxia/apraxia), and may, for example, attempt to brush their teeth with a pencil. Some people have profound agnosia (loss of the ability to interpret stimuli) and deny ownership of their affected arm, or are unable to recognise familiar faces (prosopagnosia).

Some residents may have problems finding their rooms or finding an item even if it is in front of them. There may be lack of insight into their level of abilities, difficulty with problem solving and structuring tasks. Changes of personality may have occurred that can be distressing for relatives or friends.

Key points

- After moving a resident, ensure that his or her affected limbs are well supported.
- Prevent abnormal compensatory movement patterns from occurring.
- Provide support to a shoulder joint to prevent subluxation.
- Correct positioning and 'hands-on' techniques can reduce spasticity.
- All staff should follow techniques used by treating therapists to reinforce them.
- Ask therapists about activities you can do to maximise therapeutic intervention.

Conclusion

Care staff have a substantial influence on the rate and extent of recovery after a resident has had a stroke. Care staff can help reduce spasticity and also help the psychological, cognitive and psychological problems that can ensue after a stroke by the adoption of some easy techniques. They can help improvement by following the treatment plans of the therapists and reinforce the techniques used by visiting therapists. By applying a unified approach, normal movement patterns can be reinstated and incorrect patterns of movement discouraged. They have a vital role in helping to facilitate the return of movement, reduce the effects of spasticity and prevent compensatory movement patterns developing.

CHAPTER 27

The effect of a stroke on daily living tasks

A severe stroke can cause loss of most movement patterns down one side of the body. Even with a mild stroke, difficulties can arise with daily life. Many people who have had a stroke lose the use of one hand and require help to manage daily living tasks. When part of the body is impaired (or there are sensory, cognitive or psychophysical problems), it can be frustrating for people to try to do things that they managed with ease before the stroke.

However, it is possible to use a range of different techniques to help restore some function that may have been lost and to overcome problems associated with undertaking tasks with one hand. By assisting with activities of daily living, alteration of techniques, making some minor adaptations to an individual's living space or providing assistive devices, daily living can be made easier and independence can be achieved in many activities. Each of these three approaches will be considered in turn.

Assisting with activities of daily living

It is important to find the correct balance between helping people to do a task and allowing people to do activities for themselves. Providing too much help impedes the development of independence of function: doing too little can mean individuals struggle unnecessarily. Getting this balance right is not easy and care staff can be guided by treating therapists, but the overall approach should be agreed within a care plan.

All staff should work systematically, and in a coordinated and consistent way as part of a team to achieve the plan. If this is not achieved then progress and/or maintenance of progress will be impaired.

Alteration of techniques

Following a stroke, the normal pattern of managing tasks can become seriously impeded. If arm function is substantially impaired, there is a dramatic reduction of functional abilities. This can mean that people have to unlearn the ways in which they have carried out activities over many years, and then relearn new ways of approaching things (refer to Chapter 7). It is important that this process starts as soon as possible after the stroke, to avoid people learning inappropriate ways of coping and, very importantly, to avoid the development of abnormal compensatory movement patterns. Techniques can be as simple as sitting down in order to get dressed, or using a different sequence to do tasks. Techniques are taught in conjunction with correcting posture, sequencing and encouraging use of the affected side of the body so that recovery is facilitated.

A whole sequence, such as washing, dressing or undressing, can be tiring, yet complex activities can be broken down into simple stages and each part practised. Then a sequence is built up until the total activity can be carried out. It is sensible to practice with similar items, such as cardigans and shirts, as these are put on in a similar manner. Vests, T-shirts and jumpers are also put on in the same way: the affected arm goes into a garment first and is removed last.

Minor adaptation to the environment

With some slight adaptations, rooms can be altered to make allowance for any impairment that a resident may have. If physical obstacles are minimised, there will be less need for equipment. For example: if single-action lever taps are provided to washbasins as a standard item, no tap turners or conversion to lever taps will be required. The following give some suggestions on the type of changes to the environment in care homes that can be made to minimise problems for people who have had a stroke. Further alterations to the general environment to cope with physical and cognitive impairments are discussed in Chapter 4.

■ **Entrance to room**
All homes should comply with the *National Minimum Care Standards* (Department of Health, 2003b). Standard 22.5 states that:

> Doorways into communal areas, service users' rooms, bathing and
> toilet facilities and other spaces to which wheelchair users have access,

should be of width sufficient to allow wheelchair users adequate access. In all newly built homes, new extensions to homes and first time registrations doorways into areas to which wheelchair users have access should have a clear opening of 800 mm.

Although the standards emphasise the importance of access for ambulant disabled and wheelchair users, they pay insufficient attention to many of the physical problems experienced by people who have deficits of upper limb function. As a general rule, it is helpful to go through the home checking each room with the mindset of what it might be like for a person who has had a stroke, and try to simulate their problems.

■ **Space and contents of a room**
Standard 23 states that room sizes of 12 m² should be provided for wheelchair users and 10 m² will suffice for other single users in existing homes. However, this fails to allow for the fact that some wheeled walking frames will require almost as much turning space and take up as much floor space as a wheelchair user. It also does not cater for the additional furniture belonging to a resident. Standard 34 provides a basic list of furniture, but problems may arise with access to facilities including storage of personal items.

Assistive devices

The use of assistive devices and sources is discussed in Chapter 8. The section below concentrates on specific areas that are difficult when a stroke occurs. Helpful assistive devices are suggested.

Feeding equipment and positioning

All crockery and cutlery should be within the resident's reach on a table. The chair should encourage a good sitting posture and the table should be about elbow height so that the forearms can rest comfortably on it. Dining room chairs should have armrests. There is a wide range of feeding equipment to help people who have had a stroke, including the following:

■ **Cutlery**
  – Enlarged cutlery used when handgrip is poor
  – Lightweight cutlery used when hand and arm strength is limited

- Cutlery for people with one-handed use, for example: a rounded blade with a fork at the end; a fork with one spear thickened and sharpened to provide a cutting edge; a fork, spoon and knife combined; a fork with a cutting roller on the underside

■ **Plates and dishes**
  - Plate surrounds to help with one-handed eating
  - Plates with curved edges to prevent food sliding off
  - Deep-dished plate, high-sided dish with rim or straight-sided pasta bowl to give an edge to push food up against when loading cutlery with food
  - Partitioned scoop dish
  - Suction scoop dish
  - Insulated bowls and plates to keep food warm (some have a hollow base that can be filled with hot water to keep the food warm)
  - Non-slip mats provide stability and facilitate one-handed eating

Drinking equipment

■ Cups with two handles to help people with a weak grip.
■ Clip-on straws with a one-way valve for people who are unable to suck efficiently.

Bibs and tabards

Dining bibs and tabards help to prevent food from seeping through and soiling clothing.

Cleansing and grooming

It is part of good hygiene to encourage residents to wash their hands before and after eating or toileting, if possible. It is very difficult to give your hands a good wash if you only have the use of one hand. A suction nailbrush that is attached to the sink by suction cups can be used. A perching stool or swivel seat by a basin is helpful if standing tolerance is limited or there are problems with balance or coordination.

Cleansing after toileting can be a problem and toilet roll holders that dispense only a few sheets are useful. Bathing, showering and toileting are discussed in Chapters 9-12. Even if residents require assistance to get into and out of the bath, they can be encouraged to wash themselves using a long-handled brush.

Drying bodies

Drying can be difficult, but a wash strap can be obtained or made by attaching a long piece of webbing to one end of a towel. Several manufacturers produce hand, foot and body dryers.

Dressing

If fine finger movements are impaired, then managing fastenings will be a problem. Help from others may be required or adaptation of clothing may be needed (for example, using Velcro fastenings). Clothing can be gradually replaced with clothing that is looser and which avoids intricate fastenings, such as elasticised cuffs and waistbands, open necklines and stretch fabrics. Dressing sticks, long-handled reachers, long-handled shoehorns, sock and tights aids, slip-on shoes or shoes with Velcro fastenings can help if reach and sitting balance are impaired or balance is poor.

Leisure activities

It is difficult to stabilise paper if one hand is affected. Non-slip matting can be placed beneath a thin card or a clipboard can be used. A clipboard could be kept in the office if any signatures are required, making it easier to write.

Holding a 'card' hand and playing card games is difficult, but there are some excellent cardholders available. A DIY cardholder can be made using an oblong tin and a few large elastic bands or a clean scrubbing brush turned upside down, perhaps stabilised on a piece of non-slip material.

Several leisure activities can be undertaken by using a different technique, such as sitting rather than standing to play bowls and changing hand preference. The possibilities are limitless. Residents and all staff can be encouraged to come up with suggested solutions to overcome problems.

Conclusion

Many activities are possible by altering techniques and removing obstacles within the environment; however, the use of equipment should always be considered, particularly when there are residual problems. With a little thought, life can be made easier for the residents and they can maintain and improve their level of independence.

Key points

- Many residents who have had a stroke have difficulties with activities of daily living.
- Often the alteration of a technique can make an activity easier to do.
- Provision of equipment and adaptation of the environment can achieve independence in some aspects of daily living, maintain and improve functional abilities.

CHAPTER 28

Parkinson's disease

Dr James Parkinson first described Parkinson's disease in his essay the *The Shaking Palsy* (1817). He described the cardinal symptoms as akinesia (loss of movement), a rest tremor, cogwheel rigidity and postural abnormalities. The term 'Parkinson's disease' often encompasses all clinical diagnoses falling under the broad term of Parkinson's disease. This includes Parkin Syndrome (a genetic problem) and Parkinson's Plus (which produces similar symptoms).

Gazzaniga *et al.* (2002) describe how, in the 1950s, Parkinson's disease became the first disease to be linked to neurotransmitter deficiencies. The exact cause of 'true' idiopathic Parkinson's disease, which results in a reduction in the neurotransmitter dopamine, is unknown. There is thought to be a weak genetic link, perhaps exacerbated by unknown toxins accumulating in the environment (McCall and Williams, 2004).

In 2003, it was estimated that the incidence of Parkinson's disease was 2 in every 1000 people, increasing to 1 in every 100 for elderly people and 1 in every 10 residents in nursing homes (Parkinson's Disease Society, 2003). Nazarko (2005) notes that the incidence of Parkinson's disease is rising in line with the population ageing. Parkinson's disease is one of the most common clinical groups of conditions within residential care.

Celebrities including footballer Ray Kennedy and actor Michael J. Fox have raised public awareness of the disease as they have young-onset Parkinson's disease. As knowledge of the illness has developed and professionals have gained more experience of dealing with problems and identification of coping strategies have developed.

Understanding problems

Parkinson's disease affects the initiation and performance of movement, causing stiffness and slowness of movement which progressively worsens over time. The movement pattern of the tremor experienced is similar to that of rubbing fat into flour with the fingertips, or the former pre-industrial method of making pills – hence it is termed as a 'pill-rolling' tremor. Tremor is initially present on rest, disappearing with action. People with Parkinson's disease have difficulty walking and suffer loss of balance, slow movement, poor coordination and fatigue.

Psychological problems

Although it can be difficult to determine mood because of loss of facial expression, depression and cognitive impairment are common in Parkinson's disease.

Speech

Volume, timing, articulation and pronunciation of speech can be affected, resulting in difficulty judging how a person is feeling and misinterpretation of their emotions. Speech is often quiet and may at times be inaudible or appear jumbled, simply because voice production is poor. This may be accompanied by excessive saliva production or drooling, as tongue and swallowing movements are impaired.

Scott (2005) offers tips to help when communication difficulties are present:

■ Give the person time to speak and to respond in a conversation
■ Maintain eye contact
■ Don't pretend to understand if you don't, but instead ask the person to repeat the comment in another way
■ Don't complete the end of the sentence for the person
■ Don't speak above noise
■ Use short sentences and stress key words

Scott (2005) summarises: 'Stress is easy to recognise in a person's voice, so it is important to relax. Above all, have patience and don't interrupt'.

Medical treatment

Medication remains the main treatment of Parkinson's disease. In the 1960s, many people's lives were transformed by the administration of levodopa (L-dopa), which replaced the missing neurotransmitter dopamine, providing

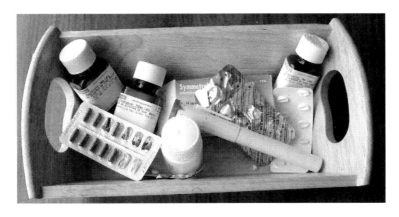

Plethora of daily medication (© NRC 2006).

major improvements to physical problems. Scadding and Gibbs (1994) noted that quality of survival has undoubtedly been improved by L-dopa treatment, although the life expectancy is still in the region of 10 years from the onset of symptoms.

McCall and Williams (2004) described how injections act as a 'rescue treatment', taking only 10–15 minutes to have an impact. An injection can be very useful when out socially, as it is faster acting than tablets, with the effect lasting for around 90 minutes. Nazarof (2005) described how subcutaneous apomorphine (Apo-go) is used to treat 'on–off' symptoms. Unfortunately, medication can result in side effects, including personality changes, hallucinations and dyskinesia (slow, writhing, jerky uncontrollable movements). Dyskinetic movements can be uncomfortable, distressing and embarrassing.

The implantation of deep brain stimulators (permanent placement of an electrode) into parts of the brain (the thalamus, the pallidum or the subthalamic nucleus) that are involved in the control of movement can help reduce symptoms such as tremor, rigidity and hypokinesia (Elias, 2005).

It should not be assumed that signs of deterioration are a natural progression of the disease; they could be related to the medication itself. It may be necessary to consult the GP or Consultant, as alterations to medication may be required. Medication therefore needs careful monitoring. In addition, some other types of medication, especially sedatives, can cause symptoms that mimic Parkinsonian symptoms. Sometimes, by simply altering medication, the symptoms can be reduced. Care staff have a vital role to play in monitoring any changes of symptoms and providing feedback to medical staff.

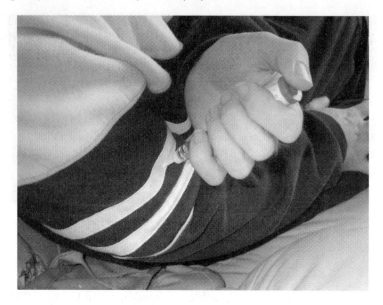

Injecting apomorphine (© Julie Swann 2007).

Problems with movement patterns

Imagine trying to perform an action but your body won't move, or wanting to smile but your muscles don't work – you would feel trapped inside your body. Many sufferers of Parkinsonism experience this. Many experience problems with walking, and balance reactions are lost.

As a result of akinesia and facial rigidity, the sufferers can look vacant and depressed. It can be very difficult to communicate with a person with a mask-like face, as there is no facial expression to interpret. Starring eyes and reduction of blinking are common.

On–off phenomenon

Some people may have periods of mobility and periods of immobility, commonly called the 'on–off' phenomenon. People may have periods of 'freezing', in which they are totally immobile, then a short period of reasonable movement patterns, followed by a period of dyskinesia (abnormal, often writhing, involuntary movements). When planning activities, it is sensible if passive activities are carried out during the 'off' period and active participative actibities encouraged during an 'on' period. 'On' periods occur about 30 minutes after

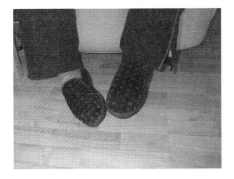
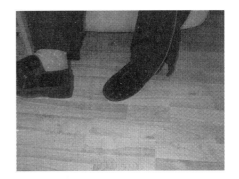
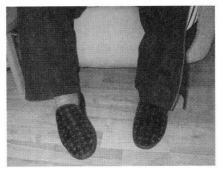

Uncontrollable dyskinesia in legs (© Julie Swann 2007).

L-dopa medication is administered. The film *Awakenings* graphically shows the effect of L-dopa on people with Parkinsonism as a result of an outbreak of encephalitis in the 1920s.

Initiating movement patterns

Initiating movement is difficult for people with Parkinson's disease and they can lack momentum when rising, for example from a chair, bed or the toilet. For older people, mobility problems can be compounded and they can literally feel stuck to a chair (start hesitation). When standing, a loss of balance can occur often due to anteriopulsion (centre of gravity is pulled forwards) or retropulsion (centre of gravity is pulled backwards) that can cause falls. This may cause the resident to move at an increasing speed to prevent falling over. Problems with stopping can arise unless a wall or chair is in their path.

Posture is often poor and shoulders are rounded (kyphotic) with the head poking forwards or held down. This posture reduces chest capacity and breathing. Walking is slow and shuffling (festinant), with loss of arm

Key points

- Parkinsonism is one of the most common clinical groups of conditions within residential care.
- Uncontrolled movements are often uncomfortable, distressing and embarrassing.
- Awareness of the side effects of medication is essential.
- Timing and alteration of techniques can optimise ability.

swinging. Residents may 'get stuck' and become 'frozen to the spot' when walking, particularly when approaching a door or chair – yet paradoxically, they can sometimes manage stairs easily.

Conclusion

Decades ago, owing to immobility, many people became bed-bound and nursing care was the main form of treatment for Parkinson's Disease. The introduction of L-dopa and subsequent medication has given increased mobility, but at a cost: major side effects include dyskinesia and 'on–off phenomenon'. Care staff must be aware of the side effects of medication and report any fluctuation in condition. Some of the impairments of cognitive function can be a result of the side effects of drugs as well as the progressive neurological damage.

CHAPTER 29

Coping with the symptoms of Parkinson's disease

Successful management of problems is important to enable individuals to participate in a wide range of social and personal situations and maintain their abilities for as long as possible. There are many ways of helping people with Parkinson's disease to re-establish an automatic rhythm, which can be applied in any situation. Techniques described here can be taught to overcome problems like initiation of movement patterns or the sense of 'freezing' that some people experience.

Strategies of coping

There are many strategies that care staff can use to help address movement problems (Tables 29.1 and 29.2). These have their foundation in the generally accepted treatment methods described in Chapter 33. Care staff can either directly assist individuals if needed, or teach residents or their relatives the different techniques. It is important, though, to make sure that a proper assessment is carried out first before intervention.

Within care, 'hands-on' care staff have the most contact with residents with Parkinson's disease; therefore they can do the most to implement activities and exercises that help with movement patterns (Table 29.2). By analysing movement patterns, parts of the day when residents are most mobile can be identified when activities appropriate to levels of mobility can be undertaken.

■ *Rhythm*

A rhythmic tune, such as a marching song, encourages automatic movements and can help overcome loss of voluntary movement. This can result in an improvement in gait pattern and also in arm swinging. Gazzaniga *et al.* (2002) describes a patient who used a stick, which he would kick to help him initiate walking by making a conscious effort.

Table 29.1 Useful techniques.

Difficulty initiating movement	Encourage rhythm by counting and then moving, e.g. 1, 2, 3, and then go
Difficulty getting up	Sit on a chair with arms of a suitable height in the lounge and dining room Bring body weight forward over knees Push on the arms of a chair to rise Use riser chairs and beds
Loss of balance	Place handrails or solid furniture strategically for support Place corner protectors on furniture, purchase future furniture with rounded corners Ensure that footwear is supportive and well fitting Arm swinging can help balance Walking equipment can provide stability if anteriopulsion is present and can bring the body forwards to prevent retropulsion Riser beds and chairs can provide a slow controlled rise to help regain balance when standing up
Posture	Encourage person to stand erect Correct posture when walking along
Getting 'stuck' when walking	Strike heel down first before moving forwards Swing the leading leg backwards and forwards before moving off Take steps back then move forwards, repeating this action if shuffling occurs March steps 'on the spot' before moving off Exaggerate movements Use visual imagery and imagination, e.g. there is a piece of wood in front that needs stepping over Twist around to look behind, then move off Instil a rhythm and encourage walking to the rhythm Practise walking to a marching song or to a distinct rhythm Count up to ten or whistle Stop, do deep breathing and relaxation techniques, then start off again
Getting stuck when going though a doorway	Use visually contrasting door strips and encourage stepping over rather than walking through a doorway

Table 29.1 (*continued*)

Steps gradually becoming smaller when walking	A carer can place a foot at right angles in front of the client's foot and encourage him/her to step over it Look ahead, not down
Tremor and dyskinesia (often increased when people are anxious)	Press arm into the body and 'fix' into this position until the tremor/dyskinesia lessens Push the feet into the floor and extend the knee Push the hands together Relaxation sessions (Chapter 20) reinforced on an individual basis

Table 29.2 How care staff can help residents with Parkinson's Disease.

- Encourage and facilitate self-management whenever possible.
- Advise on easier-to-mange clothing styles and techniques including prompting.
- Arrange for the provision of assistive equipment to help with self-care.
- Allow extra time to do tasks and concentrate on one task at a time.
- Plan daily routines around 24-hour fluctuation of function.
- Being flexible.
- Report any side-effects or changes in mobility or behaviour that may be due to side effects of medication.
- Encourage good posture and walking pattern.
- Encourage participation in social or solitary activity.
- Practice relaxation techniques.
- Reinforce input from therapists and practice exercises and activities.

Movement patterns

Part of the physical treatment of Parkinson's disease is to maintain joint suppleness and muscle power and to put a rhythm in movement patterns. Movement patterns can be practised and applied across a variety of situations; for example, reaching forwards is applied to activities like turning on taps, reaching for clothing and playing table games.

Breaking movement patterns down into small component parts and then putting these together to create a definite task-orientated movement pattern is helpful (work simplification). Movement patterns can be broken down into simple stages by experienced staff or therapists and movement patterns practised.

Encourage movements

It is important to exercise and maintain a range of movement, so ask a visiting physiotherapist for some gentle maintenance exercises. Do some specific exercises with arm swinging and leg actions in a movement to music (chair aerobics) session. Lifting legs up and down, stamping, and swinging legs and arms in time to a marching song can be practised in a seated position. 'Chair yoga' stretches help to maintain suppleness and supplement exercises.

Effect of Parkinson's disease on activities of daily living

Symptoms like bradykinesia (slow movement), tremor, akinesia (rigidity); freezing and festination (slow shuffling gait) cause problems with many daily living activities. When doing individual sessions, the emphasis is placed on individual problem areas. Specific tasks could concentrate on helping to overcome problem areas owing to impairment of fine finger movements, posture or festination. Some equipment may be required to enable a task to be carried out

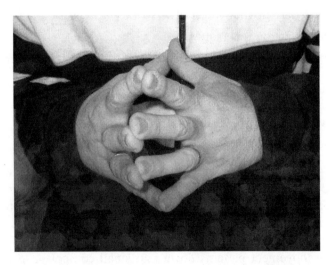

Reducing hand tremor (© Julie Swann 2007).

more easily, or indeed to achieve independence. Some useful assistive equipment is identified below and in Chapter 8.

Communication

Communication is often difficult, particularly if there is poor voice production and an expressionless face. Activities programmes could concentrate on facial movements and speech to improve expression, breathing (to assist with volume), intonation and clarity of speech. Ask a speech and language therapist about facial and speech exercises. Expression can be encouraged by activities like movement to music or games of gestures. Speech output in one-to-one or social situations can be impaired but people with Parkinson's disease can often sing. Karaoke or sing-a-longs can be enjoyable and successful activities.

Try the Conductive Education technique of using speech or inner speech to express an intention followed by movement; for example, 'I will lift up my knee' followed by the action. Use language to plan, imagine, intend and implement a movement by focusing on attention to the movement. Rhythm can be used to control the speed of the movement.

Writing

Micrographia (small writing) is a common symptom of Parkinson's disease. Try using different writing implements, such as felt tips (not as much pressure is required) or medium-nib ballpoint pens (do not show up tremor as much). Wrist weights and heavier pen enlargements may be useful. A clipboard will prevent paper from slipping. Encourage larger pen strokes.

Eating

Eating can take a long time and food may become cold if a full plate is given: try smaller portions and offer seconds. Some adapted plates have a hollow base that can be filled with hot water and sealed tightly to prevent leakage and scalding.

Fine finger movements may be difficult and enlarged handles on utensils may help. If one hand is more affected than the other, use a plate guard or straight-sided bowl with non-slip material. If there is a tremor on movement or dyskinesia, then a swivel spoon may assist to eat soups and puddings. Encourage only partial loading of food onto cutlery and try weighted cutlery.

There are many different types of drinking vessel, from ones with enlarged handles to feeding cups with spouts. Tabards are useful as they can be changed easily.

Parkinson's Disease Society (2003) state that in some people, the protein in food seems to interfere with the absorption and effectiveness of L-dopa. Doctors may suggest restricting the daytime intake of protein, but not the over-all amount of protein. Because of impairment of movement, chewing can be difficult and appropriate food (Chapter 15) should be given with a dietician's advice, if necessary.

Dressing

Several problems and solutions are provided in Chapter 13 that are relevant to residents suffering from Parkinson's disease. A gradual change of clothing style is advisable, for example elastic/stretch waistbands, slip-on shoes, and no zips or buttons. Avoid small fastenings and tight garments. Front-fasten-ing loose garments with raglan sleeves, large buttons, zips with large pulls and Velcro are easier to put on and remove. Scarves or a cravat can help if drooling is severe as they are absorbent and can be changed more easily than a top garment. If shuffling is a problem, then encourage leather-soled shoes, as these are easier to walk with and elastic or Velcro-fastened shoes are easier to manage. Natural fibres are more absorbent and comfortable to wear.

Toileting

Ensure that strategically placed handrails are available in communal toilets and *en suites*, with single-sheet toilet paper and towels within reach (Chapter 16). It may be difficult to extract toilet paper: interleaved paper may be easier, or even a box of tissues. Several manufacturers retail 'wash-and-dry' toilets. A male resident may benefit from the installation of bilateral vertical rails (to aid standing over a toilet) or a wall-fixed urinal.

Conclusion

People suffering from any deteriorating condition often meet equipment and mobility aids with resistance, as they are visible signs that activities are no longer independently possible. Therapists working in conjunction with care staff can assist to maintain function and help people to overcome areas of difficulty and prolong abilities, primarily by alteration of techniques and encouragement to use adaptive equipment.

Care workers have a critical role to play in helping ensure that people with Parkinson's disease develop techniques to enhance control of movement and learn to minimise the impact of the disease. In this way, staff can help people to move with a purpose.

Key points

- There are many techniques that can be used to minimise the impact of Parkinson's disease
- Plan activities around an individual's function if fluctuations occur from medication.
- Allow plenty of time for personal care activities to be undertaken.
- Therapeutic input and relaxation techniques can reduce tremor and dyskinesia.

CHAPTER 30

Understanding multiple sclerosis

Multiple sclerosis (MS) generally starts in early adult life and affects more women than men. In 2003, the National Institute of Health and Clinical Excellence (NICE) estimated that 'between three and seven people per 100,000 population are diagnosed with MS each year'. The Multiple Sclerosis Society (2005) describes MS as 'the most common neurological disorder among young adults, and affects around 2.5 million people in the world and 85,000 people in the UK. Every week around 50 people in the UK are diagnosed with MS. Diagnosis is usually between 20 and 40 years of age – rarely under 12 or over 55 years of age.'

Cause of MS

Although the exact cause of MS is unknown, several theories have arisen to explain why it occurs:

- Autoimmunity – the body's natural defences are actually attacking its own myelin.
- Pathogen mediated – triggered by bacteria, virii, fungi or other microbes.
- Genetic components – evidence demonstrates a genetic link.

MS therefore may result from an abnormal response to an infection or an environmental factor. Despite the lack of certainty regarding causation, much is known as to how the illness affects the body. Treatment is aimed at reducing symptoms and delaying the progression of the disease.

Effects of MS

MS attacks myelin, the protective sheath that surrounds nerve fibres within the central nervous system. Scars called 'lesions' or 'plaques' can develop in the myelin often causing damage to the actual nerve fibres. When myelin is damaged (de-myelination) the conductivity rate of the nerves slows down, leading to an accumulation of disability over time. This can interfere with neurological pathways between the brain and other parts of the body, causing distortion of messages, short-circuiting of nerve impulses or no impulse being transmitted down the nerve fibre.

As the central nervous system links all bodily activities, many different types of symptoms can appear in MS; depending upon which part of the central nervous system is affected, and the 'role' of the damaged nerve. The symptoms of MS are diverse. Jones (2006) explains, 'no two people get MS in exactly the same way and the expression of each individual's disease is as unique as their fingerprints'.

The most common symptoms and problems are:

■ Numbness or tingling in the hands or feet
■ Slowness of movement, loss of muscle strength and coordination with resultant restriction in range of movement
■ Stiffness and spasm in some muscle groups, particularly the legs
■ Balance (incoordination) and walking difficulties
■ Slurring of speech and problems articulating words
■ Difficulty swallowing and eating causing coughing and choking
■ Bladder problems including frequency or urgency of micturition sleep disturbance from nocturia (awaking needing to urinate), difficulty in passing urine or incontinence of urine
■ Bowel problems, including urgency, difficulty, pain, constipation or incontinence
■ Visual problems such as: double vision (diplopia), blurred vision (as a result of optic neuritis) and temporary loss of vision in one or both eyes
■ Dizziness
■ Pain may occur as a result of specific nerve tract involvement causing problems in a specific area, or maybe the result of muscle spasticity
■ Changes in cognitive function, e.g. loss of memory, poor concentration and slowness of thinking
■ Anxiety, depression and mood swings
■ Lack of libido, erectile and other sexual problems
■ Fatigue when attempting physical or mental forms of activity. This frequently causes difficulty or distress and can easily be mistaken for depression

Progression of MS

MS can start insidiously with no visible physical symptoms in the early stages of the disease other than: a transient numbness, a tingling sensation or slight

Table 30.1 Life expectancy after the onset of multiple sclerosis.

- In 1936, only 8% of patients were reported to survive beyond 20 years after onset of illness.

- In 1961, over 80% of multiple sclerosis patients were reported surviving to 20 years after onset of illness.

- In 2002, a patient with multiple sclerosis can expect to live to average population life expectancy minus seven years.

weakness in a limb. There may be a slight visual loss and some loss of function in one limb; or MS can cause severe functional loss, depending on the area(s) affected. People are affected in unique ways. Jones (2006) describes "MS crept up on me slowly like a boxer dancing around an opponent, weighing him up and then delivering a knockout punch". Problems with forward planning occur as a result of the variation in progression of MS and the diversity of symptoms and problems that may arise after an exacerbation of the disease. 'Predicting multiple sclerosis is like forecasting the British weather' (Jones, 2006).

The NICE (2003) guidelines on MS described three different patterns of progression:

1. **Relapsing/remitting MS** – symptoms come and go. Periods of good health or remission are followed by sudden symptoms or relapses (80% of people at onset of MS have this type of progression).
2. **Secondary progressive MS** – follows on from relapsing/remitting MS. There are gradually more or worsening symptoms with fewer remissions (about 50% of those with relapsing/remitting MS develop secondary progressive MS during the first 10 years of their illness).
3. **Primary progressive MS** – symptoms gradually develop and worsen over time (10–15% of people at onset).

Life expectancy after the onset of MS is indicated in Table 30.1 (McFox, 2002–04).

Treatment

Medication used to treat MS (Table 30.2) either treats the symptoms of MS or the underlying disease, attempting to reduce the number of flare-ups and slow the progression of physical disability. Interferons are a family of proteins naturally produced in the body that play a role in controlling the immune system and may reduce the frequency of relapses and delay the course of the disease.

Table 30.2 Medication used to treat symptoms of multiple sclerosis.

Symptom	Treatment	How this works
Relapse	Corticosteriods (methyl-prednisolone, prednisone, dexamethasone)	Shortens MS attacks by reducing inflammation in the brain and spinal cord
Muscle spasms	Muscle relaxants (Baclofen, Dantrolene, Tizanidine, Cyclobenzaprine, Clon-azepam, Diazepam)	Relieves muscle spasms to assist with movement patterns
Bladder problems	Urinary tract antispasmod-ics (Oxybutynin)	Relaxes bladder muscles and increases the bladder's ability to hold urine Reduces bladder spasms and the urge to pass urine thus lessens the frequency of involuntary urination
Pain and spasticity	Cannabis derivative (Sativex*) Oral spray	Provides relief from distressing symptoms like spasticity (stiffness and muscle spasms) and pain

*Under a 'named patient' scheme a family doctor or neurologist can write to the Home Office on behalf of the person with MS to request Sativex to be imported from Canada, where it has a license (BBC News, 2005b). Cannabis, controlled under the Misuse of Drugs Act, was reclassified to a Class C drug on 29 January 2004, although there is controversy about its use in relation to MS.

Beta-interferon is a disease-modifying therapy administered by injection. A side effect of beta-interferon treatment (Avonex, Rebif and Betaseron) can be flu-like symptoms; however, non-steroidal anti-inflammatory drugs (e.g. Ibuprofen) can reduce this side effect.

In some cases, infection may trigger a relapse; therefore people with MS should be offered immunization against influenza (NICE, 2003). Linoleic acid, 17–23 grams a day, may reduce the progression of disability and sources include: sunflower, corn, soya and safflower oils (NICE, 2003). Treatment, including stem cell transplants, is still evolving.

Emotional and cognitive effects

Coping emotionally with exacerbations and remissions can be difficult. There is a substantial amount that care staff can do on a practical level to make life easier. Psychological support may be needed. MS can profoundly affect emotions ranging from: coming to terms with the condition, fear, denial, anger, grief, depression, guilt and mood changes. The National Multiple Sclerosis Society (2005) believes that education, support, a healthy lifestyle, medications and professional help, when necessary, can make all the difference. Antidepressants may be prescribed, but NICE guidelines suggest that medication should be reviewed, if cognitive problems arise, to minimise iatrogenic cognitive losses (NICE, 2003).

Therapy can help to maintain ability and enable independence and achievement of goals and is discussed in Chapter 31.

Conclusion

MS is a progressive condition that, at present, there is no cure for; yet the treatment of MS has changed dramatically in the last decade. A more favourable outcome and better quality of life are now more attainable by people with MS by appropriate management. Drugs can be used to reduce the number and severity of MS relapses, and to reduce the number of new attacks. There is a considerable amount that care staff can do to help residents who suffer from MS.

Key points

- There is a genetic component to MS.
- Autoimmunity may be a causative factor but the exact reason for MS is unknown.
- Treatment is aimed at controlling the symptoms and preventing further damage to the myelin sheaths.
- Be alert to the onset of any speech problems and associated swallowing problems.

CHAPTER 31

Living with multiple sclerosis

Multiple sclerosis is progressive, although the rate and symptoms vary from individual-to-individual depending on which part of the nervous system is involved. Problems centre on weakness and impaired co-ordination with secondary symptoms like fatigue and depression adding to the difficulties that arise. MS is the most common cause of neurological disability in younger people and it is vital that abilities and independence are maintained for as long as possible. Physical problems cause difficulties with activities of daily living and mobility.

Activities of daily living

Independence can be facilitated in many aspects of daily living tasks. Often, the simplest solution is the most effective and also the most difficult to find. Sometimes, just by exercising creativity and flexibility, problems can be overcome. Alteration of techniques, the provision of assistive equipment (Table 31.1) and making alterations to the environment will maintain or return a degree of independence in self-care activities and daily living. Often there are several ways of dealing with the challenges that arise from impairments of function; it is important to explore all the options in order to find what is best suited to the individual. There is no ideal method of coping with a problem: we are all individuals.

Alteration of technique

Adoption of different techniques to manage tasks is often better than using, and becoming reliant on, equipment. This aspect of treatment is explored further in Chapter 7. Often a slight alteration of technique can make tasks easier and help provide transferable skills that can be used in several situations, for example:

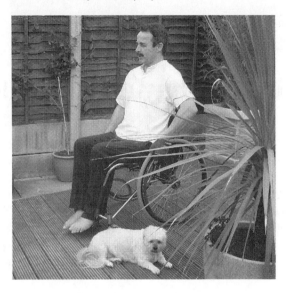

Accessible garden (© Julie Swann 2007).

- Moving from sitting to standing by 'pushing up' on thighs, rather than being reliant on the arms of a chair or a toilet frame.
- Using a waterfall technique (pouring liquids from a higher surface), when there is limited strength in the arms or impaired coordination.
- Reducing coordination problems by stabilising the elbow on the table, e.g. when feeding or writing.
- Sliding items along work surfaces, instead of lifting.

Assistive equipment

Assistive equipment and suitable mobility equipment can enable those suffering with MS to achieve a degree of independence and help to achieve some control over aspects of daily living. Some equipment may be available from the local integrated community equipment services (ICES) for individual use but not equipment that is used communally e.g. in shared bathrooms (Department of Health, 2004b). It is possible for individual assistive equipment to be obtained from ICES, e.g. for feeding or in *en suites*, but these are subject to supply (Chapter 8). Funding may be needed from the care home, the resident or their families, but many low-cost assistive devices are available from chemists or high street shops. Some homes stock general equipment to help all residents manage feeding, like: enlarged cutlery, plate guards and non-slip

Table 31.1 Small assistive equipment.

Problem area	Suggested solution
■ Feeding	
Holding cutlery because of to poor grip	Use padded, enlarged or 'L'-shaped handles
Holding cup.	Double handed cups/mugs or large 'D' handles or cups that are held with a full bilateral palm grip
Problems sucking and drinking through a straw	Use a straw with a 'one-way valve'
One-handed use	Straight-sided (pasta) bowls or plate guards Non-slip mats
■ Combing hair	
Difficulty with elevated movements because of weakness, fatigue or reduced range of movement	Long handled comb and brush
■ Writing	
Difficulty gripping pen	Try pen with larger grip Try pen with non-slip gripping surface Try rolling pins that do not need holding
Problems writing	Different type of pen, e.g. biro, medium nib fine liner Computer with either large keys or voice recognition
■ Washing self	
Unable to reach parts of body	Long handled bath brush and sponge
Difficulty standing	Sitting on perching stool or shower chair
■ Toileting	
Accessing toilets when out	Reuseable lightweight plastic urinals with lids Alter style of clothing (Chapters 13 and 14)
Cleansing self	Single sheets of paper or one-handed dispenser Wash-dry toilets
■ Wheelchair	
Propelling with sensitive hands	Wheelchair gloves

Table 31.1 (*continued*)

Poor head control	Supportive headrest
■ Reaching	
Picking up items from the floor	Long handled reacher or seat/stool/shower stool
Turning off bedside light	'Sensor' light with different light settings
■ Walking	
Unsteadiness	Walking stick, walking frame or wheeled walking frame
Carrying when using walking aid	Shoulder bag or try trolley as an alternative
Carrying when using walking frame	Clip on bag for frame

materials. Samples of small assistive equipment are provided in Table 31.1. These are also useful for many other disabling conditions.

If there is adductor spasm causing the hips to pull inwards, pommels may be useful, positioned between the legs but this can cause an increase in spasticity and contractures so will require careful monitoring.

Medication can be dispensed into easier to manage packs. Rebiject II is an auto-injector making self-injection of Rebif (beta-interferon) less painful and less complex to administer.

Adapting the environment

The external and internal environment can assist, or hinder, a person with a physical disability. Apart from the obvious access issues, e.g. level access and doorways and corridors wide enough to permit passage of a wheelchair or walking aid, other aspects need consideration. Many are discussed in Chapters 3 and 4.

Access within bedroom, en suite *and bathrooms*

Adaptation of the environment to minimise problems can be done in an unobtrusive and aesthetic manner, for example installing a higher toilet and rails rather than using a toilet frame with an integral raised seat. The environment can be rearranged so that all essential items are within reach; for example, in communal toilets toilet roll and towel holders should be within reach of an ambulant and a seated user. Mirrors should allow viewing from standing and seated positions. Cupboard doors, even with larger 'D' handles, can be difficult to access, and easy to operate sliding doors are easier to manage and enable people to be more independent. Personal grooming and clothing items could be arranged in the order that they are to be used.

Lighting and emergency call systems

Neurological problems often cause difficulties with upper limb function, resulting in loss of grip and dexterity. Rocker switches on lighting will assist and should be within reach. Sensor lights with a variety of luminance settings are useful on a bedside cabinet. Alarm cords should be within reach extending to 100 mm from the floor with a 'bangle' place between 800–1000 mm (Office of the Deputy Prime Minister, 2006). Lighting can enhance poor vision and a mirror may need task lighting, for example. Wallpaper with sheen will reflect too much light and shadows should be avoided. Fluorescent lighting tends to interfere with hearing aids.

Temperature control and sensory impairment

Extremes of temperature, like hot weather or baths, can increase symptoms, particularly fatigue. Cooling 'jackets or collars' are useful in hot weather, as are loose cotton clothes. A useful idea is to place a bottle of frozen water in front of an electric fan so that cold air is blown. Diminished sensation in the

Table 31.2 Extracts from the *Care Homes for Older People: National Minimum Standards* (Department of Health, 2003c).

Standard 25.5 states:
Pipe work and radiators are guarded or have guaranteed low temperature surfaces.
Standard 25.8 states:
Water is stored at a temperature of at least 60 °C and distributed at 50 °C minimum, to prevent risks from Legionella. To prevent risks from scalding, pre-set valves of a type unaffected by changes in water pressure and which have fail safe devices are fitted locally to provide water close to 43 °C.

hands or legs needs to be noted as a risk. Temperature control when using water is essential, otherwise there is a risk of scalds and burns. CSCI inspections require monitoring of water temperatures (Table 31.2). Extremes of temperature can have adverse effects on many medical conditions and cold can increase the perception of pain.

Management of fatigue

One of the most debilitating symptoms, particularly in the early stages of MS, is fatigue. Minor activity can trigger fatigue that impacts on every aspect of daily living. Some MS sufferers wake with an overpowering feeling of tiredness and have to rest for a while before getting out of bed, even after a good night's sleep. The following points should be borne in mind:

- Plan the day to alternate a rest or passive activity with a more active one.
- Too much activity causes fatigue, while too little can cause diminished energy, lethargy and tiredness.
- Prioritise – work out which activities are important.
- Pace tasks and perhaps do them over a few days rather than all at once.
- Simplify tasks by breaking activities into component parts with built-in breaks.
- Plan and provide frequent short rests before fatigue starts.
- Stress can increase fatigue, and relaxation techniques are useful, carried out on an individual and group basis.
- Look at the way in which tasks are performed, as ergonomics are important. An alteration of technique may assist, e.g. stabilising arms on a work surface to carry out an activity involving the hands.
- Fatigue adds to problems with speech production, coordination and mood.

Facilitating communication

Impairment of hand function causes difficulties working on a computer; word-recognition packages can help. Microsoft Windows has accessibility options including changing the size or 'blink speed' of the cursor and the display. (Go to the Control Panel's accessibility options to find out how to alter the keyboard, sound, display and mouse to allow for visual, auditory and keyboard/mouse problems). Split keyboards and ones with enlarged keypads are available. AbilityNet (http://www.abilitynet.org.uk/) specialises in assisting people with computer access problems and provides free advice to individuals.

Poor respiration produces low-volume speech or a weak voice. Pitch control can be impaired, causing an inappropriate volume of sound, and speech can sound nasal. Articulation problems result in slurred, slower speech, perhaps with long pauses between words or syllables of words (scanning speech). This may be mistaken for drunkenness.

Speech and language therapists provide guidance on how to strengthen 'speech muscles'. Care staff can facilitate speech by carrying out treatment techniques and speech practice between therapists' visits, perhaps as part of individual 'activity' time. Residents should be encouraged to talk slowly and clearly, with emphasis on intonation. Good sitting and lying posture helps with voice production and coordination. Reducing competing background noise enables a quiet voice to be heard.

Swallowing and speech problems

Swallowing and speech functions are closely interlinked. The Multiple Sclerosis Society (2004) estimates that around 50% of people with MS experience swallowing difficulties (dysphagia), although some experts report a higher figure. Furthermore, the Multiple Sclerosis Society (2004) stresses the importance of awareness of associated feeding problems that may occur as a result of MS. Problems include difficulty chewing, food sticking in the throat, sluggish movement and/or difficulty moving food back through the mouth, coughing and spluttering during or after eating and excessive saliva that causes dribbling. These can all lead to anxiety for the MS sufferer.

The Multiple Sclerosis Society (2004) notes the dangers of leaving swallowing disorders untreated, resulting in malnutrition, dehydration or even anorexia. Choking is common and has very severe consequences. Aspiration (when liquid or food from the throat goes down the wrong tube and ends up in the lungs) can be subtle and repeated chest infections may require further investigation. Aspiration can lead to infection and aspiration pneumonia. The home should have choking prevention routines and staff should be given specific first aid training to deal with choking events.

Assisting with feeding problems

If swallowing problems occur the type of food given should be easily broken up in the mouth. Enteral feeding is often considered (using the gastrointestinal tract for the delivery of nutrients). Chapter 15 provides practical ideas of how care staff can help residents with feeding problems, including chewing or swallowing foods. It may be necessary to give high-calorie snacks and nutritional drinks between meals.

There are many ways to facilitate feeding, for example:

- Encourage good posture by ensuring resident's chair is the right height and provides sufficient head and upper body support.
- Provide a relaxed atmosphere to eat that allows residents to take their time.
- Allow residents who require help with feeding plenty of time to chew food well and give time to swallow between mouthfuls.
- Alternate liquid with solid food to help the process of swallowing.
- Moisten drier foods to facilitate passage of food, e.g. by adding gravy.
- Avoid speaking and distracting residents while eating.
- Provide residents with a few sips of water between mouthfuls and after eating to remove any lingering food in the throat.
- Encourage clearing the mouth by deliberate coughing.
- Allow residents to remain upright for at least 30 minutes after the meal in order to aid digestion.

Visual problems

Although loss of visual function as a result of optic neuritis is rare, control over eye movements may be poor due to nystagmus (uncontrolled, rapid, repeated eye movements). This can be exacerbated during stress and may cause problems with reading or watching television despite the provision of spectacles; it can also aggravate difficulties with fatigue. Referral to an optometrist or ophthalmology clinic or prescribed medication may help, e.g. oral gabapentin.

Specialised equipment can be provided to assist people with visual problems, e.g. speaking or tactile clocks and watches, and large print or talking books, including those available from the Royal National Institute of the Blind.

Maintaining movement

In addition to facilitating the adoption of new techniques, care home staff can help to maintain physical function by encouraging residents to participate in activities as a means of gentle exercise. Group and individual activities can be carried out to exercise specific muscle groups in order to maintain balance, range of movement and fine finger movements. Physiotherapists or occupational therapists can devise programmes of exercises or activities.

Conclusion

It is important for those with MS to have control over their lives. Unfortunately, it is tempting to gradually do more for a resident, but this will increase their dependency on help. By looking at the problem areas, simplifying tasks, altering techniques, and providing equipment or adaptations it is possible to maintain independence for a longer period of time. And it is vital to 'do with' not 'for' those living with MS and indeed any progressive condition.

Key points

- Using a different technique can make a task easier.
- Ensuring that the design of living and communal accommodation is accessible for wheelchair and ambulant disabled users can avoid expensive adaptations.
- Assistive devices can enable activities to be carried out more easily.
- Maintenance programmes of activities are important to ensure maximum function is obtained.

PART 11

Rehabilitation

CHAPTER 32

The rehabilitation team

On admission to care many residents may have received only a small amount of NHS rehabilitation, either in the community or in hospital. There is a considerable amount that care staff can do to help residents to improve function. If a home has intermediate care beds, the home will have therapists visiting to treat residents. It is vital that care staff have a basic understanding of the principles behind rehabilitation, so that treatment techniques can be reinforced. It is important for care staff to be engaged in and familiar with treatment sessions so that they can carry out positioning, exercises or activities in between the therapist's visits to continue and reinforce treatment sessions. This is also a good way of learning and will help staff working towards NVQs. Ideas from treatment programmes can be incorporated into the resident's daily activity programme to maximise the benefit of therapy.

The rehabilitation team

The input of the primary care team (i.e. doctors, district nurses and incontinence advisors) is supplemented by rehabilitation. Physiotherapists, occupational therapists, speech and language therapists, dieticians and psychologists generally provide rehabilitation. There is also an increase in the use of alternative therapists, such as aromatherapists and reflexologists. Some homes 'buy in' private therapy or residents or their family pay for treatment. It is important that all staff are familiar with the roles of therapists and what each therapist's role is. All of these therapists should be working together and within a cohesive team, and roles will tend to overlap. Collectively, inter-professional collaboration is needed.

■ **Physiotherapists**
A physiotherapist's core skills include 'manual' (hands-on) therapy, therapeutic exercise and the application of electro-physical modalities. The aim of physiotherapy is to help the client to regain maximum functional ability and mobility through graded exercises. It is important for the resident to regain control of muscles to enable him or her to move normally, particularly after a stroke or

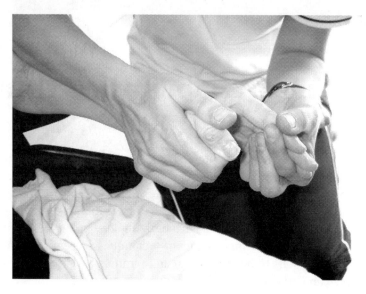

Releasing high muscle tone (© NRC 2006).

brain injury, otherwise abnormal movement patterns will result. Physiotherapy can help to prevent secondary complications and help to maintain movement and modify poor posture. Physiotherapists can help with breathing patterns, including the rate and depth of breathing and to encourage the cough reflex. The physiotherapist can provide 'chest percussion' to help bring up secretions on the lungs and prevent pneumonia.

■ Occupational therapists

Occupational therapists assess and treat people who have a wide range of physical and psychiatric conditions. Specific purposeful activity is used to prevent disability and promote independent function in all aspects of daily life. Occupational therapists maximise a person's level of abilities and independence, at the same time attempt to improve both physical and cognitive function. They can show residents different techniques to achieve independence and advise on assistive equipment for personal care activities, such as grooming, feeding and dressing. Occupational therapists can also advise on adaptations – from a handrail to help with rising, to redesigning a shower room or bathroom. They can assist the home to identify access problems and provide solutions and help to ensure many of the national minimum standards apply. Some occupational therapists provide staff training and can also advise care staff on activities to do with residents to maintain leisure pursuits. Wheelchair clinics generally have an occupational therapist in attendance who helps to identify the most suitable wheelchair for the resident and arrange for the supply of specialised supportive seating if required.

■ Speech and language therapists

Speech and language therapists will assess communication skills and provide exercises to help overcome any problems with speech. If a resident is aphasic (without speech), a pictorial 'passport' can be used. This is a book full of pictures of people, including the resident, that show his or her previous lifestyle to facilitate communication between the resident and others. Speech and language therapists can detect if a resident has control of swallowing. It is vital to ensure that the swallowing reflex is present and food goes into the oesophagus, not into the trachea (windpipe). Dysphagia (problems with swallowing) can cause inhalation (aspiration) pneumonia. In hospital, patients are often tube fed until a doctor or speech and language therapist assesses swallowing capabilities.

■ Dieticians

Dieticians can advise on a healthy diet and how care staff can maintain nutrition and hydration in residents, particularly if mastication muscles are involved. The dietician can advise on nutritious food that is easy to digest, such as thickened liquids and puréed food (Rudd *et al.*, 2000).

■ Psychologists/counsellors

Psychologists can help identify any cognitive or psychological problems that may arise from brain injuries, resulting for instance from a stroke or head injury, or dementia. After admission to a care home many people can suffer from depression and a reduction of motivation, owing to the realisation of residual disability for various reasons. Additionally, cognitive psychology may help a person come to terms with and adjust to the effects of physical or psychological problems. They can also assist in the development of coping strategies.

■ Psychiatric nurses and other specialist nursing

The community psychiatric team will provide input for residents with psychological problems. There are specialist nurses, for example continence advisors or nurses who deal with clinical groups like Parkinson's disease or multiple sclerosis.

■ Falls coordinator

This may be a nurse, occupational therapist or physiotherapist who has specialist knowledge of the reasons for falling and can help with fall prevention by identifying risk areas and obstacles within the care home environment.

■ Back care/manual handling advisor/risk assessor

Generally a physiotherapist or occupational therapist with specialist training will provide this role.

■ **Social workers**

Have a statutory duty to assess a potential resident's needs if funding for care is needed from local councils. They can offer advice, support, counselling and protection to vulnerable individuals.

Further details on other care professionals can be found on the NHS careers web site (http://www.nhscareers.nhs.uk/index.shtml).

Outline of the rehabilitation process

The broad aim of rehabilitation is to assess deficits and/or associated conditions, to identify the resident's resources and to minimise the impact on the resident's daily functional activity. Most therapists assess and treat as a continuous process a resident's abilities, and their needs can change.

■ **Assessment**

Therapists conduct their own assessments and obtain a baseline of physical and cognitive function. As roles overlap, therapists may assess and treat with another therapist from a different discipline. Assessment includes examining the range of movement and observing any alteration of muscle tone, for example decreased muscle tone (flaccidity) or increased muscle tone (spasticity). Any abnormal patterns of movement and contractures that are developing are noted. Assessment will examine sensory, perceptual and cognitive loss and psycho-social functions including alteration of mood.

■ **Goal setting**

Goals that are important to the resident are set with the therapist. Goals should be realistic and achievable, such as being able to stand up from a chair and walk two steps or to attend a community activity, for example a Sunday church service. A common approach to focus on a goal, stemming from business management techniques, is use the acronym 'S.M.A.R.T' when defining goals:

Specific
Measurable
Achievable
Relevant
Timely and tangible

SMART goals are more likely to be met and to be able to be described than non-specific, non-measurable, non-actionable, 'fuzzy' goals. To set a goal answers must be given to the following questions:

Who: Who is involved?
What: What do I want to accomplish?
Where: Identify a location or circumstance.
When: Establish a time frame.
Which: Identify requirements and constraints.
Why: Specific reasons, purpose or benefits of accomplishing the goal.

■ Treatment content

Rehabilitation tries to improve physical function and abilities. Physical therapy will concentrate initially on range of movement, stability and dexterity, rather than on muscle power. Gradually, range of movement will increase and movement patterns will become more fluid. Rehabilitation focuses on improving function by decreasing the levels of disability and handicap. Assessment and treatment work in tandem with each other.

■ Team approach

The Intercollegiate Stroke Working Party (2004) reinforce that:

> ... it is important for all team members to implement a consistent approach to rehabilitation and to maximise the carry-over outside of formal therapy, giving patients opportunity for informal practice.

Therefore, it is important for managers and senior care staff to find out which techniques are being used and to ensure that all staff and visitors facilitate therapists' techniques as consistently as possible. Therapists can provide training and clear instruction for all the staff to apply on a day-to-day basis.

Conclusion

Care staff can apply the approaches of the rehabilitation team in their everyday practice. Yet it is important to remember that no two residents are identical, and motivation is a vital key to regaining improvement. If a care home has on-site or visiting therapists, it is useful for care staff to sit in on a session or to provide sessions on activities that key workers have involvement. By learning some of the techniques, staff will be able to reinforce therapists' treatment and goals throughout a 24-hour period.

Key points

■ The roles of rehabilitation staff should be explained to care staff so that appropriate referrals can be made and inter-professional collaboration is facilitated.

■ Care staff can reinforce therapists' treatment techniques on a 24-hour basis using training and instruction provided by the therapists.

■ All people involved in a resident's care should be considered as part of the team.

CHAPTER 33

Neurological treatment techniques

Throughout life the human brain continues to be capable of learning, although the ability to learn slows down due to the effects of ageing. By using conscious cognitive and sensory pathways, it is possible to facilitate movement and maintain function.

Therapeutic treatment has changed in the past 30 years, particularly in relationship to the treatment of strokes and brain injury. Methods that were once used to attempt to improve function are now contraindicated. For example: in the early 1970s, when treating hemiplegia, patients' hands were strapped to sanding blocks and slings attached to a gantry. This supported flaccid limbs in an attempt to regain muscle power and movement. Gripping and clenching of various sized balls in the affected hand was encouraged. Unfortunately, most of these treatments only served to increase spasticity (an increase in muscle tone).

The Intercollegiate Stroke Working Party (2004) guidelines state that:

All rehabilitation approaches focus on the modification of impairment and improvement in function within everyday activities. Differences in approaches centre around the type of stimuli used and/or the emphasis on task-specific practice and/or the principles of learning followed.

Aim of treatment intervention

Following injury, the brain is capable of reorganising itself and new pathways can develop. Axonal sprouting (nerve growth) can occur and, for some, recovery may occur naturally in the first few weeks. With brain injury, this is thought to be a result of the absorption of damaged brain tissue and the reorganisation and improvement of local blood supply. The brain is adaptable, and this ability to change is termed 'plasticity'. The brain can therefore learn incorrect and correct ways of moving and can be 'moulded' as recovery takes place. It is important that after any impairment of function the brain relearns normal movement patterns, not abnormal compensatory patterns of moving. This also applies to psychophysical dysfunctions.

When treating neurological problems, several therapeutic approaches aim to direct the formation of new synapses and to open up new neural pathways or to reactivate non-functional pathways. It is important that movement is re-learned correctly; otherwise, trick movements can occur and abnormal postures and movement patterns develop, such as flexed arms, contractures and hemiplegic gait. Many techniques have evolved that are mainly based on either neurodevelopmental techniques, motor learning or relearning.

Choosing a technique

Most techniques act either by making a muscle work or by reducing or stopping muscle action. The treating therapist can show care staff how to encourage, relax or inhibit movement patterns by using techniques (Table 33.1).

It is important to realise that muscles tend to work in pairs, for example: if one muscle relaxes the other will contract, and if one muscle contracts the other will relax. This is termed 'reciprocal innervation'. Combination of techniques can produce the best results, for example, applying ice and joint compression can help release spasticity in the hand and prevent the fingers digging into the palm. This technique is useful for care staff who are involved in personal care; it can be very difficult to unclench a hand that has too much muscle tone particularly when providing hand care or washing a hand. Try placing the hand in warm water first, then apply ice (or frozen peas wrapped in a plastic bag then in a cloth) to the back of the hand for a minute to release spasticity.

Rehabilitation

Traditional treatment methods include general exercises to improve range of movement, muscle power, balance and walking patterns. Changes in practice and techniques arose as therapists gained greater understanding of the neurophysiology behind damage to the brain. Treatment has been enhanced by several specific approaches, outlined below.

■ Bobath techniques
Bobath (1990) developed techniques while working with children with cerebral palsy that are successfully used to treat stroke patients. Bobath uses inhibiting

Table 33.1 Main techniques used to inhibit or facilitate movement.

■ **Stretch reflex**

A quick stretch facilitates muscle action while a slow stretch (passive stretch) reduces spasticity.

■ **Gentle touch**

This can cause muscle groups to contract, but contraction may be delayed up to 30 minutes after application.

■ **Vibration**

1–2 seconds after application of vibration to a muscle belly, the muscle contracts.

■ **Joint receptors**

Compression of a joint, as in weight bearing through a leg, causes contraction of ankle muscles, and weight bearing through an arm facilitates activation of the muscles in the shoulder joint.

■ **Deep pressure**

This method inhibits the muscles underlying the area and encourages (excites) the opposite muscle (Bobath, 1990), and can help to reduce spasticity in an arm or leg.

■ **Ice**

The application of ice inhibits muscle contraction if it is applied to the tendon of the muscle. Application of ice to the muscle belly will cause it to contract. Ice applied to the back of the hand (muscle belly) will cause the handgrip to loosen after around 5 minutes.

---

techniques to reduce abnormal muscle tone (spasticity) and reflexes, for example putting weight through joints. Posture and head control are concentrated on. Therapists manipulate parts of the patient's body to facilitate movement patterns. Positioning of limbs is important to control muscle tone. This technique evolved into what is termed 'normal movement'.

■ **Proprioceptive neuromuscular facilitation (PNF)**

PNF is a 'hands-on' technique that reduces rigidity using active muscle contractions, prolonged stretches and auditory cues to facilitate initiation of movement (Jackson, 1998). Spiral movement patterns or diagonal movements are used and movement patterns are repeated. Therapists use 'hands-on' techniques to stretch muscle groups. All movements are reinforced by verbal commands.

■ **Rood**

Selective body positions are used that are based on the normal development of movement patterns. Sensory afferent stimuli, such as touch, stretch and pressure, are used in combinations dependent on presenting symptoms. This technique is used in the treatment of low tone (hypokinesia), slow movement (bradykinesia) or an increase in tone (spasticity).

■ Brunnstrom

Reflex activity and sensory stimulation are utilised to encourage return of movement patterns. Muscles that work together to produce a movement (synergic muscles) are concentrated on initially.

■ Conductive Education (CE)

In 1990, the Foundation for CE in Birmingham (primarily known for helping children with movement disorders), began groups for people with a stroke, multiple sclerosis and Parkinson's disease. CE is based upon intentional rhythmic movement with an approach that emphasises the need for motivation and continuity. Planned group activities are coordinated by a trained CE 'conductor'. Brown (2002) states that:

> Conductive education, like all forms of rehabilitation, does not propose to 'cure' Parkinson's. It cannot reverse neurological damage but can help control the physical manifestations of this. It offers practical techniques designed to overcome everyday problems.

■ Carr and Shepherd's approach

This approach is based on a motor relearning programme that involves practising motor tasks in their entirety. Teaching, learning and manual guidance techniques are used by therapists.

■ Johnstone's approach

This technique uses positioning and rhythmic movements in a corrective pattern. 'Air' (pneumatic) splints, made from polythene material, are applied to arms and legs to reduce spasticity (http://users.skynet.be/werkgroep. Johnstone/splint2.htm).

■ Constraint-induced movement therapy (CIT)

This technique involves restricting the use of the non-stroke upper limb whilst at the same time encouraging active use of the stroke-affected upper limb.

The Intercollegiate Stroke Working Party (2004) describes therapists using a variety of techniques to improve motor function. Stokes (1998) notes that the challenge is to be selective and innovative and not to be driven by prescription or dogma. Indeed, to date no one method of treatment seems superior to another and there is very little quantifiable difference in outcomes of neurological treatment techniques.

Conclusion

All forms of rehabilitation focus on improving function by decreasing the levels of disability and handicap. Most physical treatment aims to encourage the return of a normal movement pattern. Indeed, many care staff probably utilise some of these techniques without realising it. However, to be fully effective, it is important to understand why a resident has a physical problem, and to have a basic knowledge of what other disciplines can do to assist with movement problems.

Key points

- Treating therapists may use a variety of techniques.
- To optimise recovery, care staff should work with the treating therapists to incorporate therapeutic activities in daily routines.
- Movement disorders can be helped by simple techniques, particularly those involving rhythmical movement.

The future

The future

CHAPTER 34

Looking to the future

As the baby-boomer generations of the post-war era and the 1960s age, there is expected to be an unprecedented increase in the number of elderly people within the general population (Valeo, 2006). In the next 20 years, the number of people aged 85 and over in England is set to increase by two-thirds (Wanless, 2006). This number is projected to quadruple from 1.1 million in 2004 (1.9% of the population) to 4.2 million (6.5% of the population) in 2056 (Laing & Buisson, 2006).

Despite achieving healthier lifestyles, many people will still experience difficulties arising from physical conditions, including progressive neurological disorders, heart disease, strokes and orthopaedic problems. In addition, people with dementia and enduring mental health problems will continue to require services from statutory and private organisations. In the UK, 1.2 million people who have physical disabilities or are elderly currently receive paid-for care services (Laing & Buisson, 2006) with many people receiving additional care from friends, family and neighbours.

Evolution of services

Government policies since 1997 have affected service provision to the disabled and elderly population of the UK. *The Care Standards Act 2000 (*Department of Health, 2000) created a new regulatory framework for all currently regulated social care and independent health care services. *The Health & Social Care Act 2001* (Department of Health, 2001b) evoked changes in the structure and organisation of the NHS. Changes included integrating health and social care and provided the legal framework for the establishment of Care Trusts. Since January 2004, if a patient's discharge from acute services is delayed due to a lack of supporting community care arrangements, the culpable local authority will have to financially reimburse the relevant NHS trust.

Tightening local authority budgets means tightening eligibility criteria, only focusing on people with the highest needs. The promotion of home care includes 24-hour response teams and extra care alternatives often funded by direct payments. Several statutory and private services have evolved to enable people to live within the community rather than in long-stay institutions or care homes.

Intermediate care has provided market niches for care services providing diversi-fication and extension of service provision for some care homes, including day care and home care provision for future potential residents. Although there are now fewer places in care homes, the Government's most recent long-term population projec-tions indicate that the demand for care home places will nearly triple, from 444,000 residents in 2004 to 1.2 million residents by 2051 (Laing & Buisson, 2006).

What does the future hold?

Many changes are developing in the way the elderly care sector care is being funded. Several government policies (Department of Health, 2006a,b) outline plans for the future of care and support for older people against the backdrop of an ageing population. The Social Exclusion Unit (2006) and Wanless (2006) both provided reports on securing good care for older people in later life.

The need for services designed to cope with an increase in the ageing popula-tion will continue as people's needs, expectations and demands continue to evolve. The baby boomers (born 1945–54) are expected to object to age discrimination and to insist on greater choice and quality of care, thus presenting a cohort of more demanding social care users in the future (Wanless, 2006). People generally prefer to receive care at, or close to, home supported by respite care, day care and com-munity-based services that can provide round-the-clock care and support.

Technological advances

A new era of hi-tech products will have major impacts on our future lives: for example, telecare, mobile phones and monitoring devices.

Telecare

Telecare is defined as:

> ... the use of a combination of communications technology and sensing technologies to provide a means of manually or automatically signal-ling a local need to a remote service centre, which can then deliver or arrange an appropriate care response to the telecare service user. (Tel-ecare Services Association (TSA), 2006)

Telecare has been available in the UK for around 30 years in the form of the social alarm network. This initially consisted of a system of pull cords that were strategically sited around the home. Many pull cords were tied up as they were triggered by grandchildren, 'got in the way' or became entangled or broken. This system is gradually being replaced by body-worn alarms (wrist or pendant). Body-worn alarms provide security for elderly, frail and vulnerable people, some of whom are socially isolated or physically disabled. Around 1.5 million people in the UK currently benefit from telecare services (TSA web site). Aware of the future challenge of elderly care, the government has allocated £80 million over the next two years for telecare services with the aim of facilitating care within the person's home, avoiding the need for hospital care or care home placement.

Telecare helps to support people at home, and has the potential to postpone or prevent the need for care either at a hospital or a care home. Telecare can warn against several household risks. Smoke alarms, carbon monoxide detectors, gas alarms, low temperature alarms, flood detectors and similar warning devices can be monitored by call centres which are staffed 24 hours a day. Some monitor all local authority emergency calls, including 999 calls and people on witness protection schemes. Telecare consists of two components: specific sensors and a lifestyle package.

■ Specific sensors

Pressure or passive infrared (PIR) sensors detect movement, e.g. through a doorway, occupancy of a chair or a bed. Other examples are flood detectors, extreme temperature sensors, fall detectors, automatic lighting when getting out of bed and epilepsy sensors.

■ A lifestyle-monitoring package

Movement of items in daily use are monitored to note any changes in activity in various daily living routines, e.g. on doors (fridge, food cupboard, bed, chairs, main rooms) and electrical items (kettle, toaster, television).

Both systems are particularly useful for people with dementia or cognitive problems, 'wanderers', recent hospital discharges and those at risk of falling. Some care homes already utilise pressure pads and door sensors with residents who wander nocturnally. The device needs to be suited to the resident; for example, wanderers who are not confused will quickly learn to step over a pressure pad on the floor and therefore a bed alert or door sensor would be more suited to alerting staff.

Mobile phones

Although mobile phones are an excellent method of facilitating communication, many elderly or disabled people have difficulty operating the small buttons. To help those who might need to call the emergency services and to help locate 'wanderers', the location-tracking device (RICA, 2006) has been developed. This has a single button that alerts a call centre that relays messages to pre-programmed contacts that works beyond the boundaries of a person's home.

Telemedicine

This new technology describes medical practice across distances via telecommunications and interactive video technology. It ranges from regular medical check-ups via the Internet to high-tech microscopic 'nanorobots' capable of entering the body and repairing the human anatomy. The movie *Fantastic Voyage* (1966), an innocent science fiction fantasy, is quickly becoming reality.

Spirometric (volume of air entering and leaving the lungs) and cardiac readings can be taken in the comfort of a person's home to detect acute episodes early, thereby minimising or eliminating the need for hospitalisation. This system is currently in place for chronic obstructive pulmonary disease, cardiac and pulmonary patients in certain areas of the UK.

'Smart' clothing

Clothing containing electronic devices could act as an interface between our bodies and our surroundings. A smart shirt containing a computerised biosensor layer could monitor bodily systems, thus providing feedback or controlling the temperature of the wearer's body, for example. This would avoid the need for hands-on monitoring by staff to help to assess the overall health of individuals, although direct observation would still be required. Anderson (2005) describes how clothing could perform various functions according to individual needs and would adapt to the environment. This new era of clothing could give simple prompts reminding the wearer to take medication or to perform an activity. The implications for care provision, and for the community in general, are truly breathtaking.

Cybermedicine

Harrington (1999) described that:

> Cybermedicine sites provide a range of services, from acute medical consultations, second opinions, care for minor ailments, 24-hour,

round-the-world prescription refills, or medical referrals. Some patients appreciate the anonymity of cybermedicine, feeling able to consult about embarrassing or sensitive problems which they would not want to do face-to-face. Another advantage of cybermedicine (and telemedicine as well) is that the doctor's instructions can be printed out in hard copy for later review by the patient.... Cybermedicine's main difference from telemedicine is that there is no local doctor having face to face contact with the patient. Instead, by way of the physician's web site and/or email, the patient interacts with the cyberdoctor, conveying symptoms to the physician and receiving back a diagnosis and recommended treatment.

The future of care homes

Throughout this book, the focus has been on attention to environmental aspects. Considerable improvement has occurred in the design and interior decoration of homes. What will care homes look like in the future? Will care homes still be needed?

Standards 23 and 24 of the National Minimum Care Standards (Department of Health, 2003b) states the minimum room sizes and facilities required for single use and wheelchair users. The Single Care Home Working Subgroup (2001) describes that in Scotland and elsewhere this principle has been extended and flatlet type of accommodation with a communal lounge has been provided for residents. This allows privacy and social interaction without compromising the level of care provided or safety secured. Indeed several retirement flats already offer a domestic service and an increasing amount of personal care, if needed, with communal lounges in addition to a self-contained flat.

According to Smith (2004b) care homes are already being built with chapels, spa facilities and cinemas. Designs for future care homes will require accessible features, and will need to take dementia and dual sensory deficits into account by reducing noise, increasing the use of natural light, and providing layouts which are easy to negotiate (Smith 2004b).

Many care homes have short-stay beds that are used for respite. The NHS has purchased beds in homes to provide 'intermediate care' services that are focused on helping to restore the resident's mental or physical abilities before they return to the community. In the future, Single Care Home Working Subgroup (2001) envisages the expansion of schemes that use beds for short periods to recuperate from illness or surgery, to give people who live alone a short break or an opportunity to be 'looked after', or to provide respite for relatives who provide support and care.

Some homes provide a guest room within the care home for visitors to stay overnight. Many care homes facilitate links with schools, colleges, local clubs and vulnerable people in the community, opening social activities to relatives and friends of residents. But what about couples that want to move into a care home as a couple or indeed form a relationship within a care home setting? The media often run stories describing the emotional problems when only one partner enters into a care home. The following true case study demonstrates how needs can be met.

Case study

John and Alice, met in a residential home, and decided to marry. The home owner converted two rooms into a bedroom and lounge for them: recognising that elderly people still have a need for companionship and want to live together.

Conclusion

Technology is progressing at a rapid rate, providing benefits for people living in the community and within care homes. Tools are already available to monitor people at risk of falling and wandering who would otherwise need constant staff input.

Care homes should be seen as part of a package of care, not as a separate entity, and viewed as part of the local community. A care home has a vital role to play in the care of the vulnerable person and it is essential to adapt to the changing demands and expectations of users. Based on customer needs and wants, the future of care provision is there for the shaping.

Key points

- Technology is progressing at a rapid rate.
- Smart technology will be increasingly utilised to care for vulnerable people.
- Telecare can help within the community and care home setting.
- Care homes are diversifying and providing more community services.

CHAPTER 35

Encouraging communication through 'surfing'

Although the Internet has only been available to the public since November 1992, it has changed virtually every aspect of life in a way that could never have been foreseen. It developed from a US defence project and has become the most powerful communication tool in history, bringing with it enormous benefits – and also new dangers.

Uses of the Internet

The Internet is rapidly changing our lives. It can be accessed 24/7 from computers, televisions and some mobile phones (even when travelling). Using a wireless-free modem the Internet can be accessed anywhere in the home or garden. Access can be gained from many Internet outlets such as: Internet cafés, hotels and libraries. Using the Internet it is possible to:

- Gain instant information on millions of subjects using search engines
- Find the answer to virtually any question on any subject (useful for research)
- Watch people or observe places of interest on live web cams
- Send emails enclosing documents, digital pictures, scanned images, music, videos and voice messages
- Swap views and share information
- Hold a videoconference anywhere in the world at any time of day or night
- Play unlimited games, either solitary or against others throughout the world
- 'Chat' online and send text messages to mobile phones
- Shop or visit auction sites
- Play music and listen to the radio
- Find jobs, plan journeys, book holidays and book tickets for entertainment
- Read journals, newspapers and magazines

Around 20 years ago, these facilities were unimaginable, and 10 years ago few people saw the potential of the net. With an expanding list of uses and technology, who knows what else will be available in 10 years time?

Cyber-language

Most young people are familiar with the Internet and competent at operating computers, as the basics are taught at school. A new language swamps us. For those not familiar with terms such as dotcom, sites, surfing, emails, cyber cafés, software and hardware, there are many excellent courses. Several of the basic courses are free. Most libraries run Internet and computer 'taster' courses and provide up to an hour of free Internet use a day. learndirect (http://www.learndirect.co.uk/) provides Internet and email courses, either at local centres or online. Many staff within large statutory organisations or training within caring professions are encouraged to complete the European Computer Driving Licence Qualification (http://www.ecdl.co.uk/). The course covers using the Internet and email and can be completed online (apart from sitting examinations for the seven modules). The cost varies from centre to centre.

Sites for senior surfers

Many sites monitor demographic statistics on use of the Internet and support greater public participation by older adults. There is a growing list of Internet web sites designed to attract the active older adult – for example, Age Concern (http://www.ageconcern.org.uk/) and Saga (http://www.saga.co.uk/). 'Silver surfers' are the fastest growing group of Internet users.

Going online: cost implications

Many older people are not computer literate, but it is easy to access and use the web. Just as you don't need to understand the mechanics of a car in order to drive, it is not necessary to master the intricacies of a computer to use the Internet. With a few clicks, senior surfers can connect to relevant sites from 1p a minute to around £30 a month for broadband that provides 24-hour access, faster downloading and can include a landline package.

Modifications

Many adaptations are available to help people with difficulties access computers and the Internet. Modifications range from specialised keyboards and touch screens to hands-free operation using voice-activated commands and eye blink or laser pointers, such as those available from Keytools (http://www.keytools.com/). Abilitynet (http://www.abilitynet.org.uk/) provides online fact sheets and details of alterations that can be made to personalise a computer.

Benefits for people in a care home setting

The Internet provides both disabled and active older adults with the opportunity for instant communication throughout the world. Residents can participate equally with other generations. The Internet can reduce isolation, promote life-long learning and expand interests. Examples of opportunities for residents to take advantage of include the following:

- **Video conferences**
Real-time video and voice contact is possible with any other individual anywhere in the world. Yahoo (http://uk.yahoo.com/) and MSN messenger (http://www.msn.co.uk/) offer this facility free. Family members and friends can maintain contact with residents who live a long distance away from home, or when on holiday. Imagine the pleasure for older residents seeing their family on the computer screen when they might otherwise rarely see them.

- **Email**
Sending a message via email is easy and a good method of communicating with other computer users. Many people and businesses depend on the use of email for communication, for example for invoices, databases and marketing.

- **Text messages**
Some web sites provide free text messaging to a mobile phone.

- **Financial transactions**
Bank balances and interest rates can be obtained and money transferred across accounts. Items can be bought and sold.

- **Reducing isolation**
Global connections with people of similar interests or problems are possible using chat rooms. This is useful if no local support group is available, for

example `http://www.spinal-injury.net/spinal-cord-injury-chat-room.htm` (the spinal injuries chat room), `http://www.arthritischat.com/` (arthritis chat room) and `http://www.chatability.org.uk/` (disabled children and young people). Message board are useful means of communicating feelings and gaining information, e.g. the Alzheimer's support group (`http://groups.msn.com/AlzheimersSupport/griefboard.msnw`).

■ **Leisure facilities**

Games ranging from backgammon and chess to adventure games can be played alone or with people with similar interests.

▨ **Keeping up to date**

The Internet provides web sites on news, celebrity gossip, weather forecasts and stocks and shares, to name a few examples.

■ **Research and news groups**

Residents can find out about many subjects or share knowledge with other people with similar interests. Many companies send out regular newsletters.

■ **Recreational activities**

This can be a shared activity for residents and visitors. Visitors who are Internet literate can help the residents to contact family and friends and access sites. Places of interest can be viewed to enable informed decisions to be made as to the suitability of the venue, including the availability of refreshments and accessible toilets.

Disadvantages of the Internet

Although the Internet is a wonderful resource, it can be addictive. There are some other drawbacks, including:

■ Residents may need help from staff to access the Internet, but this can be included in individual recreational time.
■ Accuracy of information cannot be guaranteed and may be several years old.
■ Searching takes time and a trip to the library may be quicker if you are looking for a specific reference.
■ Rather than interacting with 'real' people there is a temptation to become preoccupied in solitary pursuits.
■ Chat room participants or virtual companions may not be who they appear to be. Some may prey on emotionally vulnerable people. Anonymity works

both ways; as an unknown person you can unload personal problems and yet be in control of a situation. The recipient only sees what you want to show, and vice versa. You can also be who you want to be.

■ The hunched posture caused by computer use. Providing good seating and encouraging correct posture can discourage this.

■ Eyestrain. Encourage simple measures like regular breaks from the computer.

Web sites

Web pages must be accessible for all individuals. There are many useful web sites including sites that provide hints on designing web sites for senior surfers, such as the National Library of Medicine site (http://www.nlm.nih.gov/pubs/checklist.pdf). The Spry Foundation's 36-page guide to designing web pages for older people is available electronically from http://www.spry.org/pdf/website_creators_guide.pdf. This guide also explains some of the problems of ageing that affects Internet access (Table 35.1).

The Internet can be used to locate a suitable home or services. Many homes have their own web sites and offer a virtual tour from the comfort of your own home. Details on homes can be accessed using online directories, such as http://www.bettercaring.co.uk/. Service providers can be found using directories, such as http://www.yell.com/, or key words in search engines. Full inspection reports on care homes are available from the Commission for Social Care Inspection (http://www.csci.org.uk/find_a_report.aspx).

Table 35.1 Problems of ageing that may affect Internet access. (Extracted from The Spry Foundation's *Guide to Designing Websites for Older People*)

■ **Visual problems**
  – Reduction of the field of vision
  – Difficulties following fast-moving items, such as banners
  – Problems distinguishing between light and dark
  – The perception of colour changes, causing problems differentiating between similar shades and green, blue and purple
■ **Hearing problems**
  – Understanding speech and hearing high frequencies
■ **Cognitive problems**
  – Being unable to multitask and multiprocess information
  – Becoming easily distracted by banner adverts
■ **Deterioration of motor skills**
  – Slowness inputting text into web pages when filling forms

Conclusion

The Internet continues to change the lives of many people and the impact is likely to be even greater as technology improves. Given the right level of encouragement and support from staff, residents in homes could benefit from the opportunities provided. Internet use can enhance and enrich life experiences within the care home.

Companionship and mental stimulation take only a mouse click, a keystroke or a voice command. Residents should be encouraged to enjoy surfing to complement, but not as an alternative to, face-to-face dynamic stimulation.

Key points

- The Internet opens up new opportunities for any age group in residential care.
- It is easily accessible.
- Images and documents can be transferred quickly around the world.
- The Internet can help families to stay in contact.
- Web sites are excellent marketing tools.
- Care home staff must be aware of the drawbacks of Internet use.

Glossary of main terms

Achilles tendon A tough sinew attaching the calf muscle to the back of the heel bone (calcaneus); one of the longest tendons in the body.

Ageing The process of becoming older, which is genetically determined and environmentally modulated.

Agnosia Inability to recognise everyday items. Disturbance of perception that cannot be attributed to impairments of basic sensory processed. Agnosia can be restricted to a single modality like vision or audition.

Akinesia Absence of voluntary muscular movement; characteristically seen in Parkinsonism.

Alzheimer's disease A progressive disease of the brain resulting in dementia. Symptoms include impaired memory, judgment, decision-making, orientation to physical surroundings and language problems.

Aneurysm A localised widening (dilatation) of an artery, vein or the heart. At the site of the aneurysm, there is typically a bulge and the wall is weakened and may rupture causing a haemorrhage.

Anthropometrics The measurement of the dimensions of the body and other physical characteristics.

Aphasia Language problems due to brain damage or disease (*a* = without, *phasia* = speech). Can be receptive or expressive.

Apraxia Able to recognise and describe an item, but cannot perform an action, producing difficulty carrying out skilled or purposeful movements in the absence of sensory loss or motor abnormality. Often caused by lesions in the left hemisphere of the brain.

Aromatherapy An alternative and complementary medicine based on the use of concentrated 'essential' oils from natural sources.

Arrhythmia An abnormal heart rhythm that can be too slow, too rapid, too irregular, or too early.

Arteriosclerosis Build up of plaques within the arteries causing narrowing and eventual blocking of the arteries.

Assess To judge or decide the amount, value, quality or importance of; to evaluate.

Assistive devices Any item, piece of equipment or product system used to increase, maintain or improve functional capabilities of any individual experiencing problems with activities of daily living.

Atheroma A fatty deposit in the inner lining of an artery, resulting from arteriosclerosis (atherosclerosis).

Blood–brain barrier The physical barrier between the blood vessels and the nervous tissues of the brain. This limits which materials can gain access to the neurones in the nervous system.

Botox A preparation of botulinum toxin that is injected into specific muscles to block the transmission of nerve impulses to muscles, causing paralysis. It has been successfully used in the treatment of spasticity.

Bradycardia Slow heart beats (arrhythmias)

Bradykinesia Slowness in initiating and executing movement; associated with Parkinson's disease.

Central nervous system The brain and spinal cord.

Cognition The mental act or process by which knowledge is acquired, including perception, intuition and reasoning.

Confabulation The act of describing memories of events that did not actually take place without the intention to deceive; seen in people with Korsakoff's syndrome (alcohol-induced).

Dementia A clinical syndrome encompassing progressive impairments in memory, abstract thought and judgement (executive functioning) and personality change.

Dyskinesia Difficulty with movement patterns.

Dysphagia Difficulty swallowing.

Dysphasia Difficulty with speech due to weakness and incoordination of the speech musculature.

Ergonomics The scientific discipline concerned with the understanding of the interactions among human and other elements of a system, and the profession that applies theory, principles, data and methods to design in order to optimise human well-being and overall system performance.

Executive functions The higher-level functions of the brain that produce goal-directed behaviour.

Fibrillation Irregular heart rhythm, e.g. atrial or ventricular fibrillation.

Haematuria The presence of blood in the urine.

Hemianopia Loss of half of the visual field due to brain damage; caused by injury or medical condition.

Hemiplegia Loss of function down one side of the body.

Hemiparesis Partial loss of function down one side of the body due to brain damage.

Ischaemia Impairment of blood supply to part of the body.

Intermittent claudication Pain in the legs due to impairment of the circulation of the blood to the legs; generally due to arteriosclerosis.

Long-term memory The ability to recall information over a long period, e.g. hours and days.

Multiple sclerosis (MS) An unpredictable disease causing demyelination of the central nervous system. It is marked by muscular and sensory problems causing weakness and loss of coordination. The exact problems depend on which part of the nervous system is affected.

Myelin The fatty sheath surrounding a nerve that is destroyed by Multiple Sclerosis, thus reducing the conductivity of nerve impulses.

Neurotransmitter Chemical substance that transmits a signal between neurones at nerve synapses.

Paraplegia Paralysis of the lower part of the body, including the legs.

Paraparesis Partial paralysis of the lower part of the body, including the legs.

Parkinsonian gait Stooped posture and difficulty initiating walking. Gait is festinant (short shuffling steps).

Parkinson's disease Degenerative condition that affects the basal ganglia in the brain causing a loss of dopaminergic cells in the substantia niagra. Main symptoms are rigidity, akinesia and tremor.

Plasticity The ability of the nervous system to recover after injury and to change during development.

Proprioception The process by which the body can vary muscle contraction in immediate response to incoming information regarding external forces by utilising stretch receptors in the muscles to keep track of the joint position in the body.

Prosopagnosia The abilitity to recognise faces is impaired (face blindness), while the ability to recognise objects may be relatively intact.

Reinforcement Influencing future behaviour by rewarding or punishing a particular behavioural response to a stimulus.

Selective attention The ability to focus on one subset of sensory inputs, actions or train of thoughts whilst ignoring all others.

Short-term memory The ability to retain information over seconds to minutes.

Simulation Mimicking or practising tasks.

Spasticity An increase in muscle tone.

Tachycardia Fast heart beat (arrhythmia).

Tetraplegia Paralysis of all four limbs: both arms and both legs. Alternatively called *quadriplegia*.

Tetraparesis Partial paralysis of all four limbs: both arms and both legs. Alternatively called *quadriparesis*.

Thrombosis Blood clot within the blood's circulation system.

Visual agnosia Deficits in visual perception in the absence of blindness; caused by brain damage. Person may be able to detect colours, shape and motion, but not recognise an object.

Visuo-spatial tasks Tasks involving hand–eye coordination.

References

Alkjær, T., Larsen, P. K., Pedersen, G., Nielsen, L. H. and Simonsen, E. B. (2006) Biomechanical analysis of rollator walking. *Biomedical Engineering Online*, **5**(2); http://www.pubmedcentral.nih.gov/articlerender.fcgi?artid=1334195

Alzheimer's Association (2006) *Toileting and Incontinence.* http://www.alznyc.org/_menu.main/care_prof/tips.asp#toilet

Alzheimer's Society (2004) *Policy Positions.* http://www.alzheimers.org.uk/News_and_campaigns/Policy_Watch/demography.htm

Anderson, B. (2000) *Stretching.* Shelter Publications, California.

Anderson, G. T. (2005) *Boxer Shorts that Call 9-1-1.* http://www.money.cnn.com/2005/01/13/pf/goodlife/smart_clothing/

Arthritis Foundation (2006) *Gardening & Arthritis.* http://www.arthritis.org/resources/Home_Life/gardening.asp

Aubrey-Fletcher, S. (2002) Facilitating a resident's move into a care home. *Nursing & Residential Care*, **4**(6), 289.

BBC (2006) *Create Your Own Virtual Garden.* http://www.bbc.co.uk/gardening/htbg2/virtual_garden/

BBC News (2005a) *Firms Urged to Back Design Talent.* http://news.bbc.co.uk/1/hi/technology/4272516.stm

BBC News (2005b) *Cannabis Drug Available in the UK.* http://news.bbc.co.uk/1/hi/health/4438498.stm

Barnes, M. G. (2004) *The Meditation Doctor.* Collins Brown Limited, London.

Benson, H. (1975) *The Relaxation Response.* Morrow Book Company, New York.

Better Health Channel (2005) *Gardening for Seniors.* http://www.better-health.vic.gov.au/bhcv2/bhcarticles.nsf/pages/Gardening_for_seniors?OpenDocument

Better Health Channel (2006) *Factsheet on Ageing – Muscles Bones and Joints.* http://www.betterhealth.vic.gov.au/BHCV2/bhcarticles.nsf/pages/Ageing_muscles_bones_and_joints?OpenDocument

Bo, K., Talseth, R. and Holme, I. (1999) Single blind, randomised controlled trial of pelvic floor exercises, electrical stimulation, vaginal cones, and no treatment in management of genuine stress incontinence in women. British Medical Journal, **318**(7182), 487–93.

Bobath, B. (1990) *Adult Hemiplegia: Evaluation and Treatment*, 3rd edn. Butterworth Heinemann, Oxford.

Bonner, C. (2005) *Reducing Stress-Related Behaviours in People with Dementia.* Jessica Kingsley, London.

Bosma, H., van Boxtel, M. P. J., Ponds, R. W. H. M., Jelicic, M., Houx, P., Metsemakers, J. and Jolles, J. (2002) Engaged lifestyle and cognitive function in middle and old-aged, non-demented persons: a reciprocal association? *Zeitschrift für Gerontology and Geriatrics*, **35**, 575–81.

Braver, T. S., Barch, D. M., Keys, B. A., Carter, C. S., Cohen, J. D., Kaye, J. A., Janowsky, J. S., Taylor, S. F., Yesavage, J. A., Mumenthaler, M. S., Jagust, W. J. and Reed, B. R. (2001) Context processing in older adults: Evidence for a theory relating cognitive control to neurobiology in healthy aging. *Journal of Experimental Psychology: General*, **130**, 746–63.

Brown, M. (2002) *Parkinson's and Conductive Education: PDS information sheet FS1*. http://www.parkinsons.org.uk/shared_asp_files/uploadedfiles/ {D02E182E-1289-4488-A098-985F7CA27DFD}_conductiveeducation4101_ 04.pdf

Burns, A. (2005) *Your Guide to Alzheimer's Disease*. Hodder Arnold, UK.

The Building Regulations (2000) *Statutory Instrument 2000 No. 2531 – Part M Access and Facilities for Disabled People*. The Stationery Office, London. http://www. opsi.gov.uk/si/si2000/20002531.htm

Cambridge University Press (2003) *Cambridge Learner's Dictionary*, 2nd edn. Cambridge University Press, Cambridge.

Centre for Evidence-based Purchasing (2005) *Assistive Technology Evaluation Reports*. http://www.pasa.nhs.uk/evaluation/publications/ater/

Chalfont, G. E. (2005) Creating enabling outdoor environments for residents. Nursing & Residential Care, **7**(10), 454–7.

Collier, J. (2004) *Enteral Feeding – an Overview*. http://www.dietetics.co.uk/ article_enteral_feeding2.asp

Collins (2004) *Collins English Dictionary: Complete & Unabridged*. HarperCollins, UK.

Collins, C. (2001) *Plant Alert – a Garden Guide for Parents*. Guild of Master Craftsman Publications Ltd, East Sussex.

Collins, R. (2005) *Statins 'Could Benefit Many More'*. http://news.bbc.co.uk/1/ hi/health/4282194.stm

Commission for Social Care Inspection (2005) *Inspecting for Better Lives – Delivering Change*. http://www.csci.org.uk/PDF/ibl_2.pdf

Community Care Statistics (2005) *Supported Residents (Adults) England*. NHS and Social Care Information Centre. http://www.ic.nhs.uk/pubs/comcares- rae2005/communitycarestatistics2005.pdf

The Continence Foundation (2001) *Pelvic Floor Exercises For Women*. http://www. continence-foundation.org.uk/docs/pelvwom.htm

The Continence Foundation (2005) *Disposable Body-Worn Pad*. http://www.conti- nence-foundation.org.uk/directory/subcategory.php?categoryid=70

Cowley, D. (2004) Building community ties through gardening. *Nursing & Residential Care*, **6**(7), 321.

Cressy, S. (2003) *The Beauty Therapy Fact File*, 3rd edn Butterworth Heinemann, Oxford.

Crisp, H. (2004) Preparing for inspection: a guide for managers *Nursing & Residential Care*, **6**(10), 504–6.

Crowther, M. (1996) *Traditional Massage for Health*. Parragon Book Service, Bristol.

Davies, S. and Nolan, M. (2004) Making the move: relatives' experiences of the transition to a care home. *Health and Social Care in the Community*, **12**, 517–26.

Department of Health (1992) *The Manual Handling Operations Regulations 1992*. The Stationery Office, London. http://www.opsi.gov.uk/si/si1992/Uksi_19922793_en_1.htm

Department of Health (1999) *Saving Lives: Our Healthier Nation*. Department of Health, London.

Department of Health (2000) *The Care Standards Act 2000*. The Stationery Office, London. http://www.opsi.gov.uk/acts/acts2000/20000014.htm

Department of Health (2001a) *The National Service Framework for Older People*. Department of Health, London.

Department of Health (2001b) *Health and Social Care Act 2001 – section 57 & 58*. The Stationery Office, London. http://www.opsi.gov.uk/acts/acts2001/20010015.htm

Department of Health (2002a) *Care Homes for Older People: National Minimum Standards*, 2nd edn. The Stationery Office, London.

Department of Health (2002b) *Single Assessment Process for Older People – Assessment Scales*. http://www.dh.gov.uk/PolicyAndGuidance/HealthAndSocial-CareTopics/SocialCare/SingleAssessmentProcess/fs/en

Department of Health (2002c) *How Do I Report an Adverse Incident with a Piece of Equipment? What Types of Equipment Have Been Affected Recently?* http://www.icesdoh.org.uk/faq.asp?FAQ=23

Department of Health (2003a) *Independence Matters: an Overview of the Performance of Social Care Services for Physically and Sensory Disabled People*. The Stationery Office, London.

Department of Health (2003b) *Care Homes for Older People: National Minimum Standards*. The Stationery Office, London. http://www.dh.gov.uk/asset-Root/04/05/40/07/04054007.pdf

Department of Health (2003c) *Care Homes for Older People National Minimum Standards Care Home Regulations*, 3rd edn. http://www.dh.gov.uk/asset-Root/04/13/54/03/04135403.pdf

Department of Health (2003d) *Fair Access to Care Services: Guidance on Eligibility Criteria for Adult Social Care*. Department of Health, London.

Department of Health (2004a) *Introduction to the Single Assessment Process*. http://www.dh.gov.uk/PolicyAndGuidance/HealthAndSocialCareTopics/Social-Care/SingleAssessmentProcess/SingleAssessmentProcessArticle/fs/en?CONTENT_ID=4015630&chk=MBIL%2B1

Department of Health (2004b) *Community Equipment and Care Homes*. http://www.icesdoh.org/downloads/ICES%20Equipment%20and%20Care%20Homes%2012%200ctober%202004%20-%20Main%20document.doc

Department of Health (2004c) *Community Equipment and Care Homes Appendix F: Flowcharts*. http://www.icesdoh.org/downloads/ICES%20Equipment%20and%20Care%20Homes%20Appendix%20F%20flowcharts%2012%200ctober%202004.doc

Department of Health (2006a) *Our Health, Our Care, Our Say: a New Direction for Community Services*. The Stationery Office, London. http://www.dh.gov.uk/PublicationsAndStatistics/Publications/PublicationsPolicy-

AndGuidance/PublicationsPAmpGBrowsableDocument/fs/en?CONTENT_
ID=4127552&chk=bQ7VEs

Department of Health (2006b) *A New Ambition for Old Age: Next Steps in Imple-menting the National Service Framework for Older People.* The Stationery Office, London. http://www.dh.gov.uk/assetRoot/04/13/39/47/04133947.pdf

Department of Health (2007) *The Health Benefits of Physical Activity.* Department of Health, London. http://www.dh.gov.uk/en/Policyandguidance/Healthand-socialcaretopics/Healthyliv-ing/HealthyLivingCentres/DH_4133828

Disability Discrimination Act (DDA) 1995 Part III. The Stationery Office, London. http://www.dda1995.co.uk/dda1995/theact.html

Disability Discrimination Act (DDA) 2005 Chapter 13. The Stationery Office London. http://www.opsi.gov.uk/acts/acts2005/20050013.htm

Disability Rights Commission (2002) *Policy Statement on Social Care and Independent Living.* Disability Rights Commission, Stratford Upon Avon.

Disability Rights Commission (2003) *SP7: 2004 – What it Means to You: a Guide for Service Providers.* http://www.drc.org.uk/library/publications/serv-ices_and_transport/2004_-_what_it_means_to_you_-2.aspx

Disabled Living Foundation (2003) *Choosing a Shower and Accessories.* Disabled Living Foundation, London. http://www.dlf.org.uk/factsheets/pdf/Choosing_a_shower_and_accessories_sponsored.pdf

Disabled Living Foundation (2006a) *Disabled Living Foundation Factsheets.* Disabled Living Foundation, London. http://www.dlf.org.uk/public/factsheets.html

Disabled Living Foundation (2006b) *Choosing Household Equipment.* Disabled Living Foundation, London. http://www.dlf.org.uk/factsheets/pdf/Choosing_Household_Equipment.pdf

Disabled Living Foundation (2006c) *Choosing a Bath and Bath Accessories.* Disabled Living Foundation, London. http://www.dlf.org.uk/factsheets/pdf/Choosing_a_bath_and_bath_accessories_sponsored.pdf

Disabled Living Foundation (2006d) *Clothing for Sensitive Skins* Disabled Living Foundation, London. http://www.dlf.org.uk/factsheets/pdf/Clothing_for_People_with_sensitive_skin.pdf

Disabled Living Foundation (2006e) *Choosing Toilet Equipment and Accessories.* Disabled Living Foundation, London. http://www.dlf.org.uk/factsheets/pdf/Choosing_toilet_equipment_and_accessories_sponsored.pdf

Disabled Living Foundation (2006f) *Clothing for Continence and Incontinence.* Disabled Living Foundation, London. http://www.dlf.org.uk/factsheets/pdf/Clothing_for_continence_and_incontinence.pdf

Elias, W. J. (2005) *Stereotaxic Surgery for Parkinson's Disease.* http://www.health-system.virginia.edu/internet/neurosurgery/stereotactic-surgery.cfm

Fallon-Goodhew (2002) *Yoga for Living – Stay Young.* Dorling Kindersley, London.

Finkelstein, V. (1992) *Revolution.* New Internationalist. http://www.newint.org/issue233/revolution.htm

Folliard, C. (2006) *Gentle Yoga for Health, Longevity and Rehabilitation.* Quay Books, London.

Foster, S. and Powell, J. (1992) *Gardening Ideas for Children with Special Needs.* http://extension.oregonstate.edu/catalog/html/em/em8502-e/

Fratiglioni, L., Paillard-Borg, S. and Winblad, B. (2004) An active and socially integrated lifestyle in late life might protect against dementia. *Lancet Neurology*, **3**(6), 343–53.

Gazzaniga, M. S., Ivry, R. and Mangun, G. R. (2002) *Cognitive Neuroscience: The Biology of the Mind*, 2nd edn. WW Norton & Co, New York and London.

Gipp, T. (2005) *More Tools with Shock Absorbency.* http://www.bbc.co.uk/norfolk/your/access/disability/gipp4.shtml

Goldsmith, S. (1976) *Designing for the Disabled.* RIBA Publications Ltd, London.

Goldsmith, S. (2002) *Universal Design.* Harcourt Education, Orlando.

Graham, M. (2000) *Keep Moving, Keep Young: Gentle Yoga Exercises.* Conker Productions, West Sussex.

Harrington, K. (1999) Legal implications of the practice of medicine over the Internet. Telemedicine and cybermedicine. *Cyberlaw.* 10 November, http://www.gase.com/cyberlaw/toppage11.htm

Heath and Safety Executive (2004) *Getting to Grips with Manual Handling.* http://www.hse.gov.uk/pubns/indg143.pdf

Heath and Safety Executive (2006) *Five Steps to Risk Assessment.* http://www.hse.gov.uk/risk/fivesteps.htm

Health Press Ltd (2005a) *Urinary Incontinence.* http://www.embarrassingproblems.com/urinary_b.htm

Health Press Ltd (2005b) *Urinary Incontinence.* http://www.embarrassingproblems.com/urinary_c.htm#stress

Hissey, A. (undated) *Telemedicine or Medicine and Healthcare over the Internet.* http://www.crt.net.au/etopics/telemed.htm

Intercollegiate Stroke Working Party (2004) *National Clinical Guidelines for Stroke*, 2nd edn. Royal College of Physicians, London.

International Ergonomics Association Executive Council (2000) *Ergonomics: Origin and Overview.* http://ergo.human.cornell.edu/DEA325notes/ergorigin.html

Jackson, J. (1998) *Specific Treatment Techniques in Neurological Physiotherapy*, pp. 299–311. Mosby International Limited, London.

Jacobson, E. (1938) *Progressive Relaxation.* University of Chicago Press, Chicago.

Jones, P. (2006) *What is Multiple Sclerosis?* http://www.mult-sclerosis.org/

Kent, H. (1985) *Yoga for the Disabled: a Practical Self-help Guide to a Happier Healthier Life.* Thorsons Publishing Group, New York.

Khalifah Project (2004) *Clean in Body and in Mind.* http://www.islamic-world.net/khalifah-project/Campaigns-Cleanliness.htm

Kwan, J. (2001) Clinical Epidemiology of Strokes. *Journal of Geriatric Medicine*, **3**(3), 94–8.

Laing & Buisson (2006) *Care of Elderly People UK Market Survey 2006*, 19th edn. http://www.laingbuisson.co.uk/Portals/1/contents_cepms06.pdf

Lalvani, V. (2000) *Stop the Age Clock.* Hamlyn, London.

McCall, B. and Williams, A. (2004) *Parkinson's at Your Fingertips*, 3rd edn, pp. 42–9. Class Publishing, London.

Macaulay, M., Pettersson, L., Fader, M., Cottenden, A. and Brooks, R. (2005*) Disability Assessment Report 05020: Absorbent Products for Men with Light Urinary Incontinence.* Medicines and Healthcare Products Regulatory Agency (UK).

Mace, N. and Rabins, P. (1999) *The 36 Hour Day: a Family Guide to Caring for Persons with Alzheimer's Disease and Other Confusional Illnesses* Hodder & Stoughton, London.

McFox (2002–4) *MS Facts General Information About Multiple Sclerosis.* http://www.themcfox.com/multiple-sclerosis/ms-facts/multiple-sclerosis-facts.htm

Mant, J., Wade, D. and Winner, S. (2004) Health care needs assessment: stroke. In: *Health Care Needs Assessment: the Epidemiologically Based Needs Assessment Reviews*, 2nd edn (eds. A. Stevens, J. Raftery, J. Mant and S. Simpson). Radcliffe Medical Press, Oxford.

Marshall, M. (2001) Care settings and the care environment. In: *Handbook of Dementia Care* (ed. M. A. Cantley). Open University Press, Philadelphia.

Mathias, S., Navak, U. S. and Isaacs, B. (1986) Balance in elderly patients: the 'get-up and go' test. *Archives of Physical Medicine and Rehabilitation*, **67**(6), 387–9.

Maxwell-Hudson, C. (1999) *Aromatherapy Massage.* Dorling Kindersley, London.

MedicineNet (2005) *High Blood Pressure.* http://www.medicinenet.com/high_blood_pressure/page7.htm

MedicineNet (2006) *Stroke.* http://www.medicinenet.com/stroke/article.htm

Medicines and Healthcare Products Regulatory Agencies (2003) *Medical Device/Equipment Alert – MDEA(NI)2003/25.* http://www.dhsspsni.gov.uk/niaic/mdea_updates/2003/MDEA(NI)2003-25.pdf

Multiple Sclerosis Society (2004) *Swallowing and Speech Difficulties.* http://www.mssociety.org.uk/what_is_ms/publications_shop/swal_and_spch.html

Multiple Sclerosis Society (2005) *What is MS?* http://www.mssociety.org.uk/what_is_ms/faqs/about_ms/what_is_ms.html

Murphy, B. B. (2000) *Dressing for Incontinence Care.* http://www.bigtreemurphy.com/incon.dressing.htm

Myatt, A. (2005) Part two: the history and use of aromatherapy. *Nursing & Residential Care*, **7**(8), 363–5.

National Institute for Clinical Excellence (2003) *Multiple Sclerosis – Management of Multiple Sclerosis in Primary and Secondary Care.* National Institute for Clinical Excellence, London. http://www.mssociety.org.uk/document.rm?id=271

National Institute for Clinical Excellence (2004) *Falls: Information for the Public.* http://www.nice.org.uk/guidance/CG21/publicinfo/pdf/English. National Institute for Clinical Excellence, London.

National Multiple Sclerosis Society (2005) *Emotional Aspects of MS.* http://www.nationalmssociety.org/spotlight-emotions.asp

Nazarof, L. (2005a) Part I: consequences of ageing and illness on skin. *Nursing & Residential Care*, **7**(6), 255–7.

Nazarko, L. (2005b) Causes and consequences of Parkinson's disease. *Nursing & Residential Care*, **7**(4), 158–61.

Newman, D. K. (2003) *Causes of Incontinence.* http://www.seekwellness.com/incontinence/causes.htm

Newstead, M. (2004) *A Simple Guide to Garden Planning: the Little Extras.* http://www.rhs.org.uk/advice/design/design5.asp

NHS Direct (2006a) *NHS Direct Online Health Encyclopaedia: Incontinence, Urinary.* http://www.nhsdirect.nhs.uk/articles/article.aspx?articleId=211

NHS Direct (2006b) *Statins for People with Heart Disease.* http://www.besttreat-ments.co.uk/btuk/conditions/5012.html

NHS Purchasing and Supply Agency (2005) *Improving the Life Chances of Disabled People.* Department of Health, London.

Office of the Deputy Prime Minister (2006) *Approved Document M – Access to and Use of Buildings*, 2004 edn. http://www.planningportal.gov.uk/uploads/br/BR_PDF_ADM_2004.pdf

Osborn, K. (2006) *Using Massage to Ease the Elderly's Loneliness Lifespan: Hands to Hold.* http://www.massagetherapy.com/articles/index.php/article_id/728

Parkinson, J. (1817) *An Essay on the Shaking Palsy.* Sherwood, Neely and Jones, London.

Parkinson's Disease Society (2003) *Parkinson's Aware in Primary Care.* http://www.parkinsons.org.uk/shared_asp_files/uploadedfiles/{31E42B83-775B-414F-B3C4-8708E9DC0B2C}_PDAwarePrimaryCareSept03.pdf

Patricia Neal Rehabilitation Center (2005) *A Stroke in the Family: What Can We Expect?* http://www.patneal.org/pnrc-cva2.cfm

Pavey, G. A. (1999) *Creative Gardening for Busy People.* Andre Deutsch Limited, London.

Perkins, G. O. D. (2002) *Mosby's Colour Atlas and Textbook of Neurology*, 2nd edn. Elsevier Limited, London.

Quarta, C. (2001) *Tai Chi in a Chair.* Fairwinds Press, Massachusetts.

Reid, A. (2004) Access to goods and services. *Care and Health Magazine*, 6–12 July, p. 36.

RICA (2006) *Calling for Help – a Guide to Community Alarms.* Royal Institute for Consumer Affairs, London. http://www.ricability.org.uk/reports/report-telecoms/Community%20alarms/contents.htm

Royal Association for Disability and Rehabilitation (2005) *NKS Guide – Accessible Toilets For Disabled People.* RADAR, London.

Rudd, A., Irwin, P. and Penhale, B. (2000) *Stroke at Your Fingertips.* Class Publishing, London.

Scadding, J. W. and Gibbs, J. (1994) Neurological disease. In *Textbook of Medicine*, 2nd edn (eds. R. L. Souhami and J. Moxham), p. 858–982. Churchill Livingstone, Edinburgh.

Scott, S. (2005) *Speech and Language Therapy: PDS Information Sheet.* Parkinson's Disease Society, London.

Shaw, C. (2005) *Architectural Plants.* Collins, London.

Single Care Home Working Subgroup (2001) *The Future for Care Homes in Scotland: a Consultation Paper.* Scottish Executive Consultations. http://www.scotland.gov.uk/consultations/social/fchs-00.asp

Smith, A. L. (2004a) The role of the dietician in tackling malnutrition. *Nursing & Residential Care*, **6**(1), 18–20.

Smith, C. (2004b) Bricks and mortar. *Care and Health Magazine*, 18–24 May, pp. 18–20.

Smith, J. C. (2005) *Relaxation, Meditation & Mindfulness. A Mental Health Practitioner's Guide to New and Traditional Approaches.* Springer, New York.

Social Exclusion Unit (2006) *A Sure Start to Later Life: Ending Inequalities for Older People*. Office of the Deputy Prime Minister, London. http://www.socialex-clusionunit.gov.uk/downloaddoc.asp?id=797

Social Services Inspectorate (1996) *Assessing Older People with Dementia Living in the Community: Practice Issues for Social and Health Services*. Social Services Inspectorate, London.

Stanford Stroke Centre (2006) *The Warning Signs of Stroke*. http://strokecenter.stanford.edu/consent.html

Stebbings, G. (2005) *The Year-Round Garden*. Collins, London.

The Stroke Association (2005) *The Stroke Association Annual Review 2005: The Stroke Journey*. The Stroke Association, London.

Stokes, M. (1998) *Neurological Physiotherapy*. Mosby International Ltd, UK.

Summersall, J. and Wight, J. (2004) When it's difficult to swallow: the role of the speech therapist. *Nursing & Residential Care*, **6**(11), 550–3.

Tabor, R. (2002) *All About Herbs*. Frances Lincoln, London.

Telecare Services Association (Undated) *What is a Telecare Service?* http://www.telecare.org.uk/Templates/Internal.asp?NodeID=42291

Tighe, J. (2006) *Relaxation*. http://www.bbc.co.uk/health/conditions/mental_health/coping_relaxation.shtml

Toselli, L. (2005) *A Complete Guide to Manicure and Pedicure*. New Holland Publication, London.

UK Nursing Homes Directory (2006) *The Nursing Homes Directory*. http://www.ucarewecare.com/

University of California Regents (2006) *Memory*. http://memory.ucsf.edu/Education/Topics/memory.html

Valeo, T. (2006) *Growing Old, Baby-Boomer Style*. CBS News, 10 January. http://www.cbsnews.com/stories/2006/01/10/health/webmd/main1195879.shtml

Vassallo, M., Vignaraja, R., Sharma, J. C., Briggs, R. and Allen, S. C. (2004) Predictors for falls among hospital inpatients with impaired mobility. *Journal of the Royal Society of Medicine*, **97**, 266–9. http://www.jrsm.org/cgi/content/full/97/6/266

Wanless, D. (2006) *Securing Good Care for Older People: Taking a Long-term View*, *Report of the Wanless Social Care Review*. Kings Fund, London. http://www.kingsfund.org.uk/resources/publications/securing_good.html

Weaver, D. (2005) Helping individuals to maintain mobility. *Nursing & Residential Care*, **7**(8), 343–55.

Webster, A. (1996) *Mini Relaxation Exercises*. http://www.thebody.com/mb/mini.html

Wenborn, J. (2003) Valuing music in the care home environment. *Nursing & Residential Care*, **5**(12), 574–5.

Wiebers, D. (2001) *Stroke-Free for Life*. Vermillion, UK.

Index